Conquer And Control Your Weight

Alan Fensin

Published by Burlington Books Div.
Burlington National Inc.
Box 841, Mandeville, LA 70470
United States of America
conquerandcontrol.com

All matters regarding your health require medical supervision. The ideas, procedures and suggestions contained in this book are not intended as a substitute for advice, consultation or treatment by licensed practitioners. By reading or using the information contained in this book, you are accepting responsibility for your own health and health decisions and expressly release the author and the publisher from any and all liability, loss and consequences whatsoever, including those arising from negligence.

The information in this book comes from highly regarded sources. Although reasonable efforts were made to publish reliable information, the author and the publisher assume no responsibility for the material or any consequences of its use.

Copyright © 2014 by Alan Fensin. All rights reserved. All images are copyrighted © and used with the permission of the artist. All rights reserved. No part of this book shall be reproduced, stored in a retrieval system or transmitted by any means, electronic, mechanical, photocopying, recording or otherwise, without first obtaining written permission from the publisher.

Library of Congress Control Number: 2014945822
ISBN 978-1-57706-669-9
Printed in the United States of America.

What people are saying about *Conquer and Control*

Conquer and Control isn't some feel-good, just be positive stuff. It is a logical and practical formula that you can apply to the weight problems you want to get rid of. —Joseph Keene

A pioneering and invaluable work about how to change bad habits. —Chester Imperato

This book offers indispensable practical methods to change some really bad weight problems. —Bill Malone

The *Conquer and Control* strategies are much more powerful than just using will power. Properly executed, the *Conquer and Control* principles will drastically improve your life. —Allen Brusiewski

If you want to stop an addiction, this book is invaluable. Get it and use it! —Jim Locke

Buy this book. You won't be disappointed - it will change your life. —Robert LaPierre

Fensin boils down years of eating and weight research to give us proven methods to change our destructive habits. —Bob Porter

This book takes us on a tour of our subconscious mind and shows us how to exert conscious control to change it and stop our bad habits. —Bert Phillips

Lots of books tell you what you should do, but this book shows you how to do it. —Raymond Cuomo

This is a fascinating look into the workings of the subconscious brain and how to exert control over its vast potential to control our lives. —Sam Lottel

Packed full of insights to changing bad habits, this book is well written and highly recommended. — Ed Jensen

Thank you for this book. It is a well-researched and effective way to change unhealthy addictions. This book should be required reading in every school.
—Clint Cardoza

Contents

Introduction		7
Getting Started		11
Chapter 1	Weight Control	13
	Exercise More or Eat Less	17
	Calories In	18
	All Calories Are Not the Same	19
	Sugar and Fat	24
	Sugar Substitutes	31
	Diets Radical or Slow	32
	Eating Habits, Foods to Avoid	36
	Sensible Rules	40
	Drug Side Effects	42
	Exercise	43
	Summary of Chapter	49
Chapter 2	Habit Change	51
	How Habits Work	54
	Cue, Action, Reward	56
	Beliefs	65
	Summary of Chapter	70
Chapter 3	Subconscious Mind Control	73
	Conscious Mind	88
	How to Control Subconscious	90
	PREP	92
	Seven Step Subconscious Session	98
	Summary of the Chapter	109
Conclusion		115
About the Author		117

Introduction

Congratulations on your decision to control your weight. It's amazing how many people blame society or someone else for the problems in their lives. They blame their lots in life on upbringing, family, health, bad luck, lack of money or 'the man' (usually the government or their boss). You will learn in this book that the external world does exert some influence over your habit formation, but you can regain control any time you choose. In fact, the blame game is the thing that gives you the illusion that you have less power than you really have. You can continue to blame someone else, or you can learn to take responsibility for your situations and addictions and learn how to change them. Your life can be so much easier then you imagine.

When people discover that they that they are faced with weight problems, they sometimes lose their self-respect and replace it with self-disgust or even self-loathing. When they finally learn to manage their weight over the long term, they often feel they are finally a success and their real lives have finally begun.

Major change of any kind in your life is often fearful. For many people with weight issues, the mere thought of going on a restrictive diet can fill them with fear. You may have a goal of one day losing weight, but today may not be the day. You may have previously tried to lower your weight, but after much hard work and effort failed to keep it off. Taking weight off is a combination of simple math and the desire to do it, but keeping weight off requires you to regain control of your habits.

The most important thing in achieving an appropriate weight is to make habits your friends and allies instead of your enemies and destroyers. Changing an undesirable eating or exercise habit can be very difficult if you do not understand how to do it. This is because your habits are implanted very deep within your subconscious mind. Trying to fight or resist a bad habit without knowing how often just gives strength to the habit itself. The key to changing habits is to use the methods of habit change and subconscious mind control that you will find in chapters two and three of this book.

The *Conquer and Control* method is real. It is different than anything you have tried before. If you truly want to quit your addiction, this method will work. It works because it combines the latest knowledge on habit change with state of the art technology on subconscious mind control. Taken together, you will have the tools you need to take your life back. There is nothing else like it. There is no other book like this one.

Chapter one gives you some basic information about weight, food, and exercise. It addresses the problems—both mental and physical—that an unhealthy weight can cause and provides you with the basics of how to approach those problems.

Chapter two explains how habits work. Once you understand the makeup of your life-destroying habits, you can determine which part(s) of the habit to change.

Chapter three teaches you the tools you need to use your conscious mind to reprogram your subconscious mind. You will use this reprogramming to change the habit parts you selected from chapter two.

Together, the three chapters of this book give you everything you need to change your destructive eating habit.

Of course, eating has both good and bad aspects. For example, everyone needs food, but too much is unhealthy. A good life requires enough control of your mind to adjust the factors that can lead to positive change in your life. That is what this book is about.

> You are always free to change your mind and choose a different future, or a different past. — Richard Bach

Getting Started

The book is divided into three main parts:

Chapter one clarifies the problems associated with weight and how to lose it. It explains that if you want to lose weight certain foods need to be avoided. It also explains the concept of calories in and calories out.

Chapter two explains why we have habits and the best way to change these habits.

Chapter three is about controlling your subconscious mind. Often we need extra help to change a habit. Our subconscious mind is very powerful and is able to assist us in changing stubborn habits.

Chapter One
Weight Control

> Don't dig your grave with your own knife and fork. — Proverb

Eating is usually pleasurable, but it has the power to enslave you. It can become your master and destroy your ability to live a long, healthy life. Food addiction can be just as powerful an addiction as drugs, cigarettes, alcohol and all the rest of the addictive life-destroyers. In some ways, food addiction is worse because we all need to eat a normal amount of food to live. We can avoid drugs and most other addictive substances and activities, but food is all around us and constantly available. We can't just say no to food because we need it every day. Some days it's special, such as on Halloween where I recall how much fun it was going to strangers' homes as they gave me bags full of sugar products to eat.

Over 200,000 years ago when food was scarce, our bodies evolved into a sophisticated life form that endeavored to store enough extra fat to keep us alive. Hundreds of years, ago there was a certain prestige in being overweight. Back then, hunger and food shortages were normal and periodically threatened survival. In that time, an overweight person obviously came from a well-off family and was seen as having status in their community.

But today in America, food is everywhere and even a very poor person can be extremely overweight. There are even candy bars and sugar soft drinks in unsuspecting locations such as Home Depot. Today, being overweight is recognized as a health hazard, and instead of prestige it is considered a sign of weakness. In fact, more than half a million Americas needlessly die each year because of unhealthy diets and insufficient exercise.

You may believe the slogan, "eat, drink, and be merry, for tomorrow we die." But if you eat too much, tomorrow will come sooner than you think.

> Inside some of us is a thin person struggling to get out, but they can usually be sedated with a few pieces of chocolate cake.
> — Unknown

Freud theorized that the first organ to emerge as an erotogenic zone is the mouth. From the time of birth onwards, the baby's psychical activity is concentrated on providing satisfaction with the mouth for nourishment, peace and pleasure. As adults, many of us still use food as a relaxing drug that provides peace and a release from loneliness and many other problems of life.

However, with this release, we also take on increased risk for a number of very bad diseases. These include diabetes, high blood pressure, heart disease, cancer, liver and gallbladder disease, respiratory problems, osteoarthritis, and others. It's not surprising that studies have shown a significantly higher mortality rate for overweight people. In America, about thirty percent of people are considered obese.

We all know that our body is irreplaceable, yet many people are not aware of all the dangers of obesity. Now you know, and it's never too late to begin regaining your health.

Chapter One Weight

> I'm not overweight. I'm just nine inches too short. — Shelley Winters

There is a genetic component to being overweight. Genetics cause some people to be tall and some short. It causes some people to easily build strong muscles while others will be weaker. Some people store fat in their belly and others in their rear end, legs, et cetera. Some people are smart, and some people are not as smart. Some people have a full head of hair, and some are hair free. Some people have higher metabolisms and others lower. So it should not come as a surprise that some people just naturally have a fatter or leaner body. If you pay attention, you can see that body shape often runs in families. A small percentage of people have an underactive thyroid that can slow down their metabolism and contribute to weight gain. Some people even have extra copies of genes for digesting carbohydrates from grains. The perfect weight for you will be different than the perfect weight for someone else.

Regardless of genetics, you can still lose weight if you really want to. You can create your own destiny, but some people have to work smarter and harder than others. But depending on your genetics, you may never be able to have the skinny, emaciated look of some models.

The main obstacles to losing weight are long term behaviors and habits that must be changed. However, most people cling to their existing habits and resist change. This book gives you the **CAR** habit control and the **PREP** subconscious control tools to work smarter and beat weight problems. You will find these tools in chapters two and three. They are very effective in changing many bad eating habits.

16 Conquer and Control

> My doctor told me to stop having intimate dinners for four unless there are three other people. — Orson Welles

Many grocery store checkout lines have racks filled with women's magazines touting various eating regimens that claim to magically melt your pounds away. These can work temporarily, but the problem with them is they are all based on will power, which typically is unsustainable.

It seems there is a new fad diet at least every month. Some books will tell you to eat a high carbohydrate diet and others will recommend a low carbohydrate diet. Various authorities have recommended eating margarine instead of butter, but years later they say eat butter instead of margarine. My mother used to say that liver is better to eat than meat, but now most scientists say that liver is not as good as meat. Like most people, I gave up following the ever-changing diet fads and stayed with my same old diet, but still found it harder and harder to keep the weight off.

> I've been on a constant diet for the last two decades. I've lost a total of 789 pounds.
> — Erma Bombeck

There are many thousands of books written about how to lose weight with some quick fix. You might have tried some but had no lasting results. The key here is "lasting," because even though you lost one pound a day for three weeks, you then gained it all back again. Any diet that says to eat less calories will help you lose weight, but trying to stay on one of these diets using willpower alone is difficult and usually does not work. Additionally, going on and off the diet of the month is actually harmful to your body and you typically gain weight in the long term with rollercoaster diets. As one comic said, "I keep trying to lose weight but it keeps finding me."

The number one reason that your willpower usually fails to keep the weight off is that you've become addicted to sugar and refined carbohydrates. Eventually, the sugar withdrawal symptoms become too much for your willpower and you go back to your old eating habits. Regrettably, after falling off your quick fix diet, you may blame yourself and feel like a failure. Our goal in this book is to use habit changes and subconscious mind control to successfully lose weight slowly and keep it off.

> Dieting is not a piece of cake. — Unknown

Exercise More or Eat Less is Simplistic

Calories Out

It seems obvious that if you burn more calories than you consume you will lose weight. In reality, there is a lot more to it. The concept of joining a gym or club will definitely burn the calories. However most people find that they do not ending up losing weight. You need to burn 3,500 calories to lose a pound of fat. If you exercise for an hour, you are lucky to burn one ounce of fat.

There are numerous reasons to exercise regularly, and everyone should exercise. It may not, however, help you lose weight. Exercise improves self-image, fitness and longevity. It reduces heart disease, diabetes and various other health issues. For weight loss, increasing exercise burns more calories than a sedentary life. Unfortunately, it usually has the effect of increasing your appetite, which neutralizes the weight reduction effects of calories out. Most of us can attest to the fact that after a day of vigorous physical activity, we are famished and seek a big meal.

Before beginning a routine of greater physical activity, you must first use habit change techniques to resist increasing your caloric consumption. I do recommend that you establish a regular routine of aerobic exercise as a part of your weight loss. Ideally, you should do at least thirty minutes of some form of exercise at least four times a week. This can be something as simple as walking or any exercise strenuous enough to raise your heart rate. Other ideas include swimming, using machines at the gym, or almost anything as long as your body is moving. But you must not increase your caloric intake if you want to lose weight. There is more on exercise at the end of this chapter.

Calories In

The other side of the coin is dieting to decrease caloric intake. Here there are two things to be aware of that have the potential to trip up your goal of losing weight.

First, by drastically limiting your calorie intake, you put your body into survival mode so you will not starve to death. Your body automatically reduces its metabolism so now you have reduced your calories out as well as calories in. Fortunately, your metabolism returns to normal after a few weeks of regular eating.

The end result is that the long-term difference

between calories in and calories out may not change much. The solution is to use habit change techniques to increase physical activities. Just thirty minutes of exercise can increase the resting metabolism for the next thirty hours.

You may temporally lose weight with drastic food restrictions, but there are few people that can live their life that way. When our old eating habits return, people put the weight back on, and often more due to the fact that your now-reduced metabolism is storing fat for your next survival challenge. Also, in addition to the fat loss from a drastic diet you also lose much muscle. So after returning to your old eating habits you end up with less muscle and more fat.

If it were just the balance between calories in and out, there would not be the need for so many books, and America (along with some other countries) would not be having such a huge obesity problem. The recommendation to eat less and exercise more is logical, but it has not worked for most people. Willpower alone is not enough to stop the urge to eat more. As much as you try, most people cannot stop thinking about food or get that urge to eat out of their head.

> In general, mankind, since the improvement of cookery, eats twice as much as nature requires. — Benjamin Franklin

All Calories Are Not the Same

The second thing to be aware of is that all calories are not the same. For example, calories from protein consumption are different than calories from refined sugars. The reason for this is that sugar in your blood (glucose) will increase certain hormones, such as insulin. Insulin works to store the energy from sugars and increase fat deposits in our body.

A self-preservation function of our bodies automatically saves nourishment in the form of fat to keep us alive during times of scarce food. While most of us no longer are in danger of starving to death, our bodies are genetically preprogrammed to keep us alive. For example, bears that hibernate in the winter eat many fattening foods in the fall to increase their fat content during the long winter days of sleeping in their cave. I remember kayaking in Alaska's Inner Passage and watching bears strip the fatty skin from fish and throwing the rest of the fish away. These bears are the ones who lived to reproduce and pass this survival trait to their offspring. (A side note here is that cold water fish fats such as salmon, sardines, whitefish, tuna, rainbow trout and mackerel are very high in omega 3 oils, which are much better for our bodies than fats from land animals or hydrogenated vegetable oils.)

> A waist is a terrible thing to mind.
> — Tom Wilson

While shopping at grocery stores we are often unaware of the sugars in things like salad dressing, alcoholic beverages, and sports drinks. Canned foods such as fruit, applesauce, soups, and dried fruit often have significant amounts of sugar added. Likewise, our body quickly converts some starches such as potatoes and corn into sugar. Often the names of the ingredients are misleading. For example, the term corn syrup or fructose is used instead of sugar even though they both taste sweet and both produce glucose in our body. Corn syrup is even worse than sugar. The average American diet is dominated by refined carbohydrates, and this is the number one reason our waists are so big.

So the solution here is to replace the refined sugars, corn syrup, refined grains, et cetera with fruit, vegetables, protein and whole grain products. The reason is that sugars and refined grains enter the blood stream so quickly that our body, to process them, produces more of the hormones that increase our fat. When the sugars are still contained within their fibers, their release is much slower and they do not do the damage of the refined carbs.

Additionally, eating foods with more fiber can speed up the movement of the digestive tract, ending up in quicker disposal of the foods. This gives food less time to put their calories into the blood stream. Fiber also seems to reduce the occurrence of colon cancer and diverticulitis. Fiber can also soak up fat in the stomach, keeping it from being absorbed into your body. Additionally, fiber adds bulk to food without additional calories thus giving you more of that full and satisfied feeling. Fiber comes from vegetables, fruits, and whole, unrefined grain. You can also add more pure fiber you can buy from many grocery stores or online. This fiber is actually the part of the grain or rice that is removed during the refining and milling process.

> When I buy cookies I eat just four and throw the rest away. But first I spray them with Raid so I won't dig them out of the garbage later. Be careful, though, because Raid really doesn't taste that bad.
> — Janette Barber

The National Institute of Health says that excessive sugar and fructose consumption is linked to diseases such as hypertension, type 2 diabetes, liver disease, heart disease, and Alzheimer's. They have created the glycemic index, which measures how quickly glucose (sugar) rises in your blood after eating various foods. Pure sugar is the worse and causes the body to produce a lot of insulin. Unrefined carbohydrates take much longer and put less glucose in the blood. They have a lower glycemic number and produce less insulin as well as put less fat on your body.

Another reason that refined carbohydrates puts the pounds on is they enter your system so fast that your body has no choice but to turn them into fat. The unrefined carbohydrates enter your system more slowly and your body has the time to use them up for energy without storing them as fat.

The glycemic index ranks carbohydrates on how quickly they are broken down and how they affect your blood sugar. Refined carbohydrates such as white bread and sugary food are absorbed much quicker than unrefined carbohydrates. They cause a rapid rise in blood sugar and produce fat in your body. When food is quickly digested and causes rapid blood sugar rise it is given a high glycemic index.

High (bad) glycemic index foods include refined foods such as white bread, corn chips, most sugars, bagels, Kaiser rolls, candy, watermelon, baked white potatoes, refined cereal such as Total, Cheerios, Corn flakes, Rice Krispies, sports drinks, sugary drinks, ice cream, et cetera.

Low (good) glycemic index foods include unrefined grains and vegetables, dark and unsweetened chocolate, brown rice, beans, peanuts, most meat, et cetera.

The lists above just have the basic information. There are many thousands of foods, but the main thing to remember is that processed foods generally have a higher glycemic index than unprocessed foods. For information on other foods, check the internet and type in "glycemic index foods." You can also consult one of the many books on the glycemic index.

So the bottom line here is to replace certain calories with different calories in order to lose weight. This book recommends a balanced approach by taking all of the factors, including habit change, into account. You do not have to eat less, but you have to eat different things.

> The point to keep in mind is that you don't lose fat because you cut calories; you lose fat because you cut out the foods that make you fat-the carbohydrates. — Gary Taubes

The concept of eating lean cuts of meat and cutting excess fats off your meat is still relevant. Even though sugar is worse for you than fat, I do not mean to imply that eating a lot of fat is ok. An ounce of fat has more than twice as many calories as an ounce of protein.

Saturated fats and trans fats (hydrogenated) have been shown to contribute to many diseases such as cancer, strokes, artery disease, and more. The meats our hunter–gather ancestors ate were very lean. They came from wild animals that that had to run to survive, so they were much leaner than the meats we buy today at at the grocery store. Our modern animals were selectively bred and fed foods that made them grow faster and fatter than the wild animals and fish that our ancestors consumed. Fat is not as bad as sugar, but it is still bad so trim the fat and eat less fat and butter. Vegetable oil consumption should also be reduced but not eliminated. Saturated (bad) fats to be eliminated include palm and coconut oils, dairy products (except for skim and low fat products), margarine, et cetera. Meat products such as beef, pork, lamb, and chicken should be trimmed to reduce the fat as much as possible.

Sugar and Fat

Some prescription drugs can affect your metabolism, often causing significant weight gain. Among them are insulin, steroids, anticonvulsants, antipsychotic drugs, and antidepressants. Normal body hormones also affect your metabolism and play a role in why you gain weight. One example is that young women who have a lot of estrogen have some protection against gaining weight, but when they get older and estrogen decreases, more fat often accumulates in their fat cells. Testosterone shifts have the same result in older men.

Even how you eat can change your metabolism. Three meals a day is healthy. However skipping breakfast and lunch causes your body to begin survival mode and lowers your metabolism. Then when you eat a large dinner more of the food turns to fat.

Of the few dozen hormones that regulate our body weight, insulin is by far the most important. When carbohydrates (especially refined carbohydrates like sugar and white flour) are eaten, they end up in our blood as glucose. Our pancreas then makes more of the insulin hormone to control the blood lever of glucose. The insulin triggers the body to store the glucose throughout the body in various cells. Some glucose goes into fat cells to be stored for periods of famine, which for most people in America never comes.

> Sometimes I had difficulty remembering that "all you can eat" is not a personal challenge. — Marika Christian

When our blood glucose and insulin levels decrease, our body will use the energy stored in our fat cells to keep all the body functions active until the next meal. However, if we get a lot of calories from refined carbohydrates, our body will still have a high level of insulin and instead of getting energy from our fat cells, we will get hungry and eat more food. This causes us to gain more and more weight and often results in the various health problems of obesity. Additionally, high levels of insulin cause your body to become insulin resistant. Then your body needs more insulin, and when your pancreas produces it it causes your body to store yet more fat. Another problem is that insulin resistance often results in type two diabetes.

Type two diabetes is associated with excessive refined carbohydrate consumption. It begins with a condition called insulin resistance. This is where insulin receptors do not recognize insulin and will not bind with it. This causes high levels of glucose in the blood. Your pancreas cannot keep up with the increased demand for insulin and results in too much glucose in your blood. If left untreated, serious life threatening diseases occur.

For about the last two hundred thousand years (depending on how you define humans), we have been hunter/gathers with a diet of meat, fish, nuts, roots seeds, fruits and various plants. During those thousands of years our bodies evolved to help us survive with the foods available to eat. Consuming both animals and plants resulted in better nutrition and larger brains.

For the early humans, none of these foods were processed. Depending on their location, sugar from fruit was only available to our ancestors for a few months a year. During the winter months their diet had less plants and more meats. For those hundreds of thousand of years, the humans that did best on these foods passed their genetics on to their children. Over time our genetics have been optimized for these types of food. It's only during the last few hundred years that large amounts of processed foods such as white flour, white sugar, white rice, et cetera, have been abundantly available to most people.

In processed (refined) foods, the fiber and the germ (the living part of grain) are removed and the sugars and starches remain. Our bodies have not genetically adapted to these new processed foods, so it is not surprising that they cause health problems. And the problems are getting worse. In 1973, Americans were eating about 45 pounds of sugar annually and less than 2% of Americans were diagnosed with diabetes. By 2010 they were eating 77 pounds of sugar and diabetes increased to 7%. And it is even higher today.

Added sugars in your food

12 oz. soft drink	36 grams of sugar
10 oz. milkshake	36 grams of sugar
Three cookies	24 grams of sugar
One slice cake & frosting	24 grams of sugar
One cup sweet breakfast cereal	12 grams of sugar

As societies began producing and eating more refined carbohydrates, the incidence of obesity also increased. So it is the association of refined carbohydrates with production of the insulin hormone that is responsible for most of the weight gain. In a very small percentage of the population, some other hormones and genetics affect our weight gain. However, in most cases, the cause of weight gain and diabetes is the ingestion of refined carbohydrates that triggers the body's production of insulin.

For all of human existence earth has been in our current ice age, which periodically gets colder or warmer. (Our current ice age is called the Pliocene-Quaternary, and it started about 2.58 million years ago.) Only twelve thousand years ago, most of North America, Northern Europe, and other areas were covered by ice over two miles thick. And because the water was tied up in ice, the oceans were an amazing four hundred feet lower than they are today. It was only in the last eleven thousand years that the earth moved to one of its warming periods. During the colder periods there was less plant growth so humans had to rely much more on hunting animals and less on gathering plants. Fortunately, our bodies adapted to survive on either plant or animal food.

Different people are affected by carbohydrates in different ways. During the two hundred thousand years of human existence, the gatherers (who lived closer to the equator) developed a higher tolerance for carbohydrates then the hunters. However, neither group evolved enough to deal with today's highly refined sugars (such as the high fructose corn syrup found in today's soft drinks and elsewhere).

Sugar is literally an addictive drug. It produces dopamine and stimulates the pleasure centers of the brain much like heroin does. If you have a sweet tooth, you will find that keeping a normal body weight is difficult. But with the help of this book it is possible and it must be done.

Carbohydrates, when they are refined, make us

fat. The bottom line of any diet must be to get rid of refined carbohydrates. This takes a conscious effort because many products have sugar added to make the food taste better. Also, many fat-free items have added sugar. Even the American government USDA dietary guidelines recommend that we choose foods and beverages with little added sugars or caloric sweeteners.

> Bigger snacks mean bigger slacks.
> — Unknown

Artificial sweeteners make many foods taste better. However, if you are still addicted to sugar, the substitutes will not end your craving; you will have the strong desire to eat another item to relieve your sugar desires.

In all honesty, at first I personally had difficulty with this low refined carbohydrate concept. However, I accepted the scientific facts and it worked for me. It will also work for you.

> Broccoli might get stuck in your teeth, but French fries will get stuck in your thighs.
> — Unknown

There is no absolute number of how many carbohydrates we can eat and still lose weight. Humans are all different, but one thing is certain: if you're overweight, your current level of refined carbohydrates consumption is too much and contributes to your obesity.

So how does one proceed? First you should consider starting a moderate exercise routine. This may be as simple as walking three times a week. The goal here is to begin feeling better about yourself by moving around and promoting better circulation in your body. Again be aware that your exercise may cause an increased appetite. We recommend it because everyone, regardless of weight, should have some exercise. If you do not have the will power to do some type of regular exercise then use the information in chapters one and two and create a habit. If you cannot walk very far, walk as far as you can and increase it over time. If you cannot walk at all, get a few small weights and work with them at home, or join a gym and use some of their equipment. Read more on exercise in the last section of this chapter.

> The second day of a diet is always easier than the first. By the second day, you're off it. — Jackie Gleason

Next comes the type of foods you eat. If you can simply change your diet in one fell swoop and stick to it, then do that. However, as the expression goes, people often bite off more than they can chew. If you are unsure, then just try it and watch the results. If it doesn't work, you will have to take it slower. If you can't just stop, then reducing slowly will still work. Pick one of the items you consume, such as sugary soft drinks, and replace them with unsweetened tea or coffee, or just plain water. Then after a few weeks, choose another item to put on your do not eat list. This will take you longer then the crash diets, but you will be more likely to have long-term success.

If you still have difficulty, then just start with something that you can more easily give up. Giving up one can of soda a day is the minimum way to start. The following chapters will teach you how to program your subconscious to do that.

As you get more experience at programming

your subconscious habits, you will find it easier to give up those soft drinks. Once you have lost your excess weight, then you can decide on which food items to allow back into your diet. The goal is to eventually give up all of the refined carbohydrates. After you succeed in this goal you will have lost weight and you will keep it off.

You may have been on some diet, lost some weight and then gained it all back. You may think it is impossible to lose weight and keep it off. If you just use willpower to control your eating, you probably will gain the weight back. But I am here to tell you that changing your subconscious habits to reduce your refined carbohydrate consumption is different. It will let you lose weight and keep it off.

Take a look at these before and after pictures of Bob. He changed his subconscious habits, gave up refined carbs, and exercised regularly. Now he looks like a different person. I didn't include his picture to show that he lost a lot of weight. I included his picture because the weight is never coming back. He went from 240 pounds to 185 pounds about ten years ago, and because he changed his subconscious habits, the weight loss is permanent and he will not gain it back.

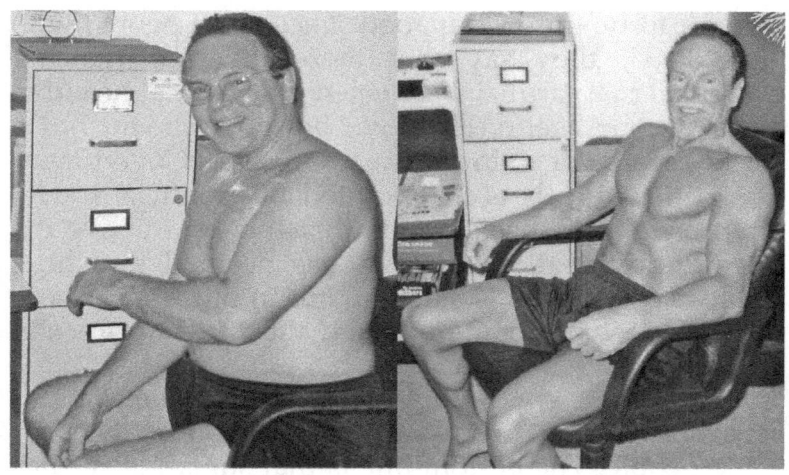

Sugar substitute safety

Ideally you can just give up your sugary drinks and drink water or unsweetened beverages such as unsweetened tea or coffee. But many people have to give up sugar in steps, and these people often switch to "diet" drinks first and then to water or unsweetened tea. However, about one hundredth of one percent of Americans have a condition called Phenylketonuria (PKU). These people should definitely not take sugar substitutes such as aspartame (Equal, NutraSweet, et cetera) that came out in 1981. Another problem is that for some people, artificial sweeteners slow down their metabolism, and that of course means they burn less calories then they would have if they just drank completely unsweetened drinks. But for most people, artificial sweeteners are a great stepping-stone to reducing their sugar intake while they use habit change to eventually not need any sweeteners.

Of course aspartame (like anything relatively new) has not been around long enough to definitively call it safe. The FDA has deemed that aspartame is safe enough to be put in our food. Except for people who have PKU, they say that there is no convincing evidence that artificial sweeteners have a negative effect on our health. However big government has a track record of lying to us citizens. Government department heads are appointed by politicians who often have a political agenda that they put above the truth. Additionally, the FDA has deemed that high fructose corn syrup is safe enough to put in our food. So in the case of sugar and sugar substitutes, we really don't know what is true and what is just politics.

We do know that our body metabolizes aspartame into toxins, which can cause problems for some people. The bottom line is that sugar substitutes have problems and should not be called safe. However, if you are overweight and have diabetes in your family, and don't have PKU, then aspartame is safer than sugar and especially high fructose corn syrup. However, the best course of action is to stay away from both sugars and artificial sweeteners and drink water or beverages with no sweeteners in them.

Diets – Radical or Slow

An example of a fast radical carbohydrate restrictive diet is the Atkins diet. This type of diet requires huge changes in the food you eat. If you have the willpower to stay on this type of diet, that's great, but you are in the minority. Using the habit control ideas in chapters two and three will help tremendously. Food is so prevalent in our society that the constant temptations can easily challenge our resolve. Also, if you go on a fast, radical diet, you should check with a professional to be sure you are not pre-diabetic. Some people have died when the rapid change in their blood sugar level caused them to lose consciousness.

We prefer to take a more long-term view and slowly change our diet. This means changing our habits slowly enough so our body gets used to the sugar reductions. This is important since, as I stated earlier, sugars act like a drug that stimulates pleasure parts of our brain. With some drugs—such as opiates—a total abstinence is recommend. But with sugar, the habit control in the next chapter and slow but steady reduction work best for most people. Additionally, your cravings for sweet food will diminish after you begin to eat less of it.

> Inch by inch, anything's a cinch.
> — Robert Schuller

What works is the reduction of those processed foods such as sugar and starches. Complex carbohydrates such as broccoli release their glucoses more slowly and do not create a huge insulin reaction from the pancreas. Also, the fiber from these natural foods is necessary to healthy functions of body. Various research studies concluded that people who eat whole grains that are high in fiber weigh less than those who eat less refined grains.

We are all different so it is up to you to determine which foods in your diet to begin reducing. If you usually have three dinner rolls with your meal, cut down to two. Don't bring the third to the table to tempt yourself, either.

If you drink a sugar drink with your meal, switch to water. If you can't switch to water with no flavor, then at least you can change to an unsweetened drink. The concept is that, with your daily work on habit control from the next chapter, you will have the power to easily give up one or two things. Then after a few weeks you can reduce another item. It might be another dinner roll or that cola you drink in the afternoon, or that candy, or that sugar in your coffee. Remember that your health and very life depend on decreasing your refined carbohydrates consumption.

Do not continually ask yourself if you are losing weight or achieving your goals. Weigh yourself regularly but remember body fluids can easily increase or decrease your weight by ten or more pounds. Naturally, you want regular, quick results. But give your subconscious mind time to manifest those results. It is counterproductive to seek new results every day or even every week. The largest trees grow from a small seed, and that seed may be in the ground for many months before sprouting and beginning its growth.

All goals should be framed in positive terms. For example, "I do not want to be fat," will not work as well as, "I have a normal looking body," or, "My normal weight is now 130 pounds."

> A overweight person doesn't eat what's right but eats what's left. — Unknown

Many overweight people are emotional eaters. They eat to escape from something in their lives. That may be boredom, intimacy fear, depression, frustration, anxiety, stress, pain, exhaustion, relationships, or any number of similar emotions. This need to escape often drives people to gorge on food. Addressing all of your emotions is a difficult and time-consuming task, so instead this book uses habit change and mind control to alter your habits so you can find comfort in something healthier, like unrefined carbohydrates or something besides food. Examining your habit cycle **CAR** (from chapter two) will provide some self-awareness necessary to change your lifestyle. What are your personal **C**ues, **A**ctions, and **R**ewards from eating? You probably know what some of these habit cycles are without much thought. These would be the ones to start with.

Ask yourself if you are hungry. Are you someone that eats not because you are hungry, but for some other reason (like comfort)? If you are not physically hungry, ask yourself why you want to eat. Pay attention to what intense emotional reasons drive you to eat. Food is an enjoyable way to forget our feelings. It is often said that we figuratively eat our feelings. If this is you, pay attention to the emotional cues that instigate your hunger.

> Gluttony is an emotional escape, a sign something is eating us. — Peter De Vries

Compulsive eating often comes from instructions to "clean your plate" or similar programming that became habits. It usually was installed in our subconscious mind during our childhood, but today it still controls us.

Metabolic hormones have a large influence on your metabolism and its ability to burn calories or store fat. There are literally hundreds of hormones in our body, and a few of them, such as adrenaline, can either raise or lower our metabolism. This is one reason that aging, which reduces many of these hormones, often results in weight gain for those who eat similarly to the way they did when they were young.

Exercise can increase our fat-burning hormones, and their effect on our body can last for up to thirty hours after we finish exercise. This keeps our metabolism higher and is effective in reducing fat. However we should not forget that regardless of our metabolism, the old rule is still true: to lose weight, you must eat fewer refined calories than you burn.

Numerous studies have shown that slowly reducing calories—especially refined carbohydrates—and exercising regularly is a very effective way to lose weight and keep it off. Depending on your age and condition, the exercise can be very moderate (such as walking) or more vigorous (such as playing tennis or other sports). The main component is regular, meaning at least three times a week.

Everyone has to eat, and for the obese person each occurrence of normal hunger may be a powerful cue to eat to excess. If it is a cue for you to overeat, then this is definitely one of the cue-triggered habits for you to modify.

When you do the seven step subconscious sessions that are in chapter three, visualize yourself as having already conquered the bad habit you had. What are you doing now that you lost eighty pounds, look great, are in control of your life, and have much more energy? Use your imagination to make this picture vivid and real and your subconscious will endorse what you believe and make it your reality.

> He who cures a disease may be the [most skillful], but he that prevents it is the safest physician. — Thomas Fuller

Eating Habits

Below are some examples of various types of eaters and possible ways to proceed. Your eating habits may be different than these examples, but you can use similar techniques. You may also have more than one eating habit that you use on various occasions.

Comfort eaters get emotional relief from their food. Food can numb the pain and be a source of comfort and solace during times of stress. You may have grown up with the saying "eat something; it will make you feel better." Now if you're frustrated, sad, bored, angry, lonely, anxious, et cetera, you eat. The cue here is the emotional problem and this is not easy to change. For example, you may be angry with your boss but unable to find a better job, so you feel stuck and you use sugar to temporarily "fix" the problem.

The action is what and how you eat, and you can modify this. Less sugar and refined carbohydrates and more vegetables and meats would still give you the reward of comfort. Another modification of the action would be to eat more slowly; it takes about 15 minutes for you to become aware that you are full, so eating more slowly often means you eat less overall.

If your cue is not physical hunger, then some other action could be performed to get a similar reward. The reward, of course, is the comfort you feel when you are eating. Determine your hunger cues by examining the main types of eaters listed below:

Hunger eaters may have just completed hard physical work, exercised at the gym, et cetera, and their body actually needs the nourishment. This is true hunger and not just eating due to your desire. You can't change the cue but you can change the action. As with the comfort eater, less sugar and refined carbohydrates and more vegetables and meats would still give your body the nourishment it desires.

Social eaters eat with their family or friends and lose track of how much they eat in the comradeship during the meal. Or you may habitually eat everything to please the hostess. You may also have various subconscious habits from childhood, such as always cleaning your plate.

Pleasure eaters love to eat because they believe the taste and smell of their gourmet food is pleasurable. Pleasure eaters consider themselves connoisseurs of good food and drink. But in addition to treating their taste buds, they are also feeding their sugar addiction. Their cue is the recurring thoughts of delicious fine foods. They could modify their action and eat gourmet food with less sugar and refined carbohydrates and more vegetables and meats. They would still get the same reward.

Automatic eaters do not pay attention to their food when they eat while watching television or even while driving.

Compulsive eaters can't seem to stop eating refined carbohydrates and often keep their home stocked with bags of chips, soft drinks, cookies, cakes, et cetera. Often they begin eating without any conscious thought to the matter. Their sugar addiction is the cue, and similar to other strong addictions it is not easily broken. The action can be changed by replacing the unhealthy snacks in their homes with healthy ones (such as fruit).

Reprogramming your subconscious to desire an apple more than a bag of chips and a soft drink could change the reward. To do this, review **PREP** from chapter two. In this instance you can repeat a few times a day that you will eat an apple when you have an urge to eat. Attach love to your thoughts on apples and picture yourself slowly enjoying eating the delicious apple.

Various studies show that people who drink water, sugar free tea, coffee or eat soup before their meal consume fewer calories. This is because the liquids fill you up, causing you to eat less when the food comes.

> After exercising I always eat a pizza...Just kidding I never exercise. — Unknown

Below is a list of foods to avoid. Remember, do not change your diet all at once, because few people can make drastic changes without a relapse. To have a sustainable diet, make one small change at a time. It may take you a year to avoid all these foods. Start out with sugar and fructose. Take a few months to give up all of the forms, such as soft drinks, donuts, ice cream, candy, desserts, and the other various sweets you eat or drink.

Foods to Avoid

- **Sugar** including fruit juice and high fructose corn syrup.
- **Processed carbohydrates** including white flour, white rice, potatoes, sugar, starches, jam, candy, soft drinks, pasta, white bread, cookies, cake, pie, ice cream, et cetera.
- **Potatoes and other starches** including french fries, sweet potatoes, corn, watermelon, pumpkin, and bananas.
- **Hydrogenated oils** including margarine.
- **Excessive animal fats** (trim fat from your meat).
- **Excessive vegetable oil** (use less). Additionally, people with certain conditions may want to avoid salt, milk products, artificial sweeteners and gluten.
- **Fruit juice**, but most whole fruit is ok.
- **Replace the avoided foods with:** fruit, vegetables, nuts, whole grains, beans, fish and

lean meats. Also take a good multi-vitamin and mineral pill every day.

You should monitor your progress, so weigh yourself about once a week, but don't make the scale your only appraisal of success. With a changed diet, fluid retention and loss will cause significant weight changes. In addition, if you are exercising more then your new muscle will actually weigh more than the same volume of fat. Other things to take into account are your energy level, your blood pressure, how your clothes fit, and other measurements such as your cholesterol levels. Remember that the weight loss process is not straight up. There are hills and valleys, but have patience and you will win.

Sensible Rules

- Eat fewer refined carbohydrates and fats.
- Do not drink your calories. Sugary drinks to not satisfy your hunger as well as solid food.
- Eat a large breakfast and a small dinner.
- Eat three meals a day.
- Do not skip meals.
- Never eat fewer than two hours before bedtime.
- Stop eating if you feel full.
- Get tempting foods out of your home.
- Pay attention to your eating and minimize distractions.
- Take smaller bites of food.
- Chew slowly and take longer to eat in order to feel satisfied on less food.
- Don't watch TV while you eat.
- Don't eat quickly. Slow down and you often eat less.

- Eat a smaller supper and a larger lunch.
- Weigh yourself at the same time of day to minimize fluid retention changes.
- Drink a large glass of water before every meal. It will fill you up faster, and you need more water during periods of weight loss.
- Take a multi-vitamin and mineral pill every day. This will stop any cravings for vitamins you may be missing.
- Eat only while seated at a table and not while doing something else.
- Eat vegetables to help you feel full.
- Eat an apple every day.
- Chewing sugar free gum can substitute for food and calm you down. Chewing is an instinctive habit and with gum, you also end up eating less food.
- In addition, chewing your food longer satisfies your chewing instinct so you eat less.
- Eat healthy salads with low fat dressings.
- Fill up on vegetables and fruits.
- Don't go on drastic diets that you will probably quit in a few weeks.
- Track the number of calories you eat for a week to see where you can cut back.
- Don't snack on junk food between meals.
- Don't skip meals.
- Not all brown bread is 100 percent whole wheat. Check the ingredients.
- A glass of beer or wine has about the same glucose content as a slice of cake.

- Think before you eat, but if you are physically hungry and not emotionally hungry, eat something nutritious.
- Skip the dessert after your meal.

There are refined carbohydrates in many items that at first you might not think about. Almost all fruit juices have the plant fiber removed and are now basically fructose, which raises your insulin level just like other sugars. Any foods made from white flour—including most breads—is missing the fiber. Many items have added sugar for taste, including many breads, frozen dinners, and cereals. White rice has the fiber striped away. Potatoes are almost all starch with little fiber.

> It's 2014 why does food still have calories...
> —Unknown

Some authors claim that certain blood types can handle carbohydrates better than others. For example, type A is supposed to handle carbohydrates better than type O. This sounds good and may be true, but I couldn't find any proof in my research. It still might be true, however, since genetically some people do handle carbohydrates better than others.

Drug Side Effects

Some prescription drugs can affect your metabolism and interfere with your ability to normally lose weight. Anti-depressants can affect your weight, so check with your physician to be sure you are taking the correct medicine at the lowest effective dosage. Steroids also can cause weight problems. Pain medication that comes from opiates can be an issue as well. This does not mean that you can't lose weight, but you should be aware that you might have to consume even fewer calories than you would if you weren't taking the medication.

> Whether you think you can or think you can't, you are usually right. — Henry Ford

Exercise

> Whenever I feel the need to exercise, I lie down until it goes away. — Paul Terry

Earlier in this chapter I said that the concept of exercising more to lose weight is simplistic. That is because exercise increases your appetite. Most people would feel justified in eating more since they just lost all of that weight with the exercise. Also, if you want to lose weight, reducing refined carbohydrates trumps exercising because it is considerably more efficient at reducing calories.

In fact, lowering your refined carbohydrate calories consumption is about three times more effective than increasing your calories burned through exercise. Still, a combination of both works best, which is why I added this final section on exercise.

But there is still another reason I concentrate on eating instead of exercise. That is because most people who need to lose weight will not form a regular exercise habit; at least, not until they start seeing their weight coming off from reducing their intake refined carbohydrate calories. Running an 8-minute-mile is a great aerobic exercise and calorie burner, but I am sure you're not going to do it. But you might start out walking or working out on an elliptical machine, treadmill, or a regular or stationary exercise bike.

If you don't want to go to a gym, you can often get good prices on used equipment. Some of the equipment is compact and folds down to fit under your bed or in a small storage room.

It's a fact that many people who will easily go on temporary but very restricting diets will not even remotely consider regular exercise. But there are many kinds of exercise, and chances are that one of them can be right for you.

> If it weren't for the fact that the TV set and the refrigerator are so far apart, some of us wouldn't get any exercise at all.
> — Joey Adams

Depending on your current condition, there are many types of aerobic exercise that you can do. If you have not exercised for a very long time or are really out of shape, you should definitely consult a physician before starting.

Swimming targets many muscles in your body and is also a great aerobic exercise. If you can jog, you will burn a lot of calories. Jumping rope is good for younger people with strong knees. Bike riding can also burn a lot of calories. Additionally, many of these exercises can be done inside on treadmills or stationary bikes. And one of the easiest is just walking.

If you think you can't possibly do any type of regular exercise, check out chapter three. I know there are many excuses people use to continue doing the same old thing, but you can use subconscious mind control to override the natural objections your subconscious mind throws out to avoid change in your life.

> An early-morning walk is a blessing for the whole day. — Henry Thoreau

At the gym I go to, January is a very busy month. Following their New Year's resolutions, many people join the gym and obligate themselves for one year of membership dues. But they only last a month or two before their willpower runs out and they rationalize they have more important and pressing things to do with their lives.

Difficult aerobic classes and weights are certainly not for everybody. Furthermore, using some of those exercise machines without training can even be dangerous. Many people go to the gym for vanity exercise to build up certain muscles they believe look good on them. That is fine if it's what you want, but our goal in this book is to use aerobics to assist you in losing weight and generally getting in shape.

> If there had been an exercise I'd liked, would I have gotten this big in the first place?"
> — Jennifer Weiner

Once you take control of your eating habits, regular exercise can be an important part of weight loss. Exercise can reset your metabolism to help you burn more calories. In addition to increasing your metabolism to help control your weight, regular exercise can reduce your risk of diabetes, heart disease, high blood pressure, and even joint and back pain.

> Walking is the best possible exercise. Habituate yourself to walk very far.
> — Thomas Jefferson

The American Heart Association has thoroughly researched the results of physical activity. The AHA recommends that adults should be physically active for at least two and a half hours per week. If you walk vigorously for half an hour or more each day, you exceed these recommendations.

Any type of exercise is good and burns calories, but you'll burn more calories with aerobic exercise than with strength and resistance exercise. Consequently, for someone who does not currently exercise, the easiest exercise to start with is simple walking. I recommend a good pair of running shoes, even though you are only walking, but walking shoes or any shoes can start you out.

Some forms of exercise are very good but can't be done everywhere. For example, swimming can really burn calories, but you need a pool. And even if you always have access to a large enough outdoor pool, most people would not want to swim in the winter. Not so with walking.

While walking, you should swing your arms to increase the value of the exercise. Keep a good posture: upright and with your shoulders back. If you can, walk vigorously or eventually work up to a vigorous walk. After your initial warm-up period, you want to walk quickly enough to break a sweat. You also want to keep sweating for the entire time of the exercise.

If necessary, you can start out with just five minute walks where you obviously won't break a sweat. Eventually, however, you need to build up to at least half an hour a day of brisk walking. But don't get over-motivated and push yourself too hard for your physical condition.

Walking is my main exercise. I like it because

there is no special equipment needed except some proper shoes and a hat for the sun. On trips I can walk and see some new scenery at the same time. At home I enjoy walking around a nearby park. It is surprising how many people I meet during my walks. It is also soft on my knees, which is important at my age.

I have found that it is best to walk at the same time every day so you develop a habit of doing it. Some people prefer a bicycle instead, which also works well. The concept is to get your heart and lungs going in order to reset your metabolism and get your body to start burning more calories. And the American Heart Association says you will also live longer.

I walk in the early morning because it establishes a habit. In the cold winter I use an indoor machine, but some people go to the local indoor mall and walk there. Other people go to a gym and use their machines. The most popular for those trying to lose weight are the elliptical machine (which is gentle to your knees) and the treadmill. Next in popularity seems to be the spin classes, which are stationary bikes that a group rides at various intensities to simulate outdoor scenes. Other people like rowing machines, which exercise both the lower and upper parts of your body.

It is good to have an exercise friend or partner. This keeps you going since it is more than just you. Walking and talking is typically much more fun than exercising by yourself.

> To reduce your weight, turn your head to the right then to the left. Repeat every time you are offered fattening food to eat.
> — Unknown

People have various physical limitations, but almost everyone can do some sort of regular exercise. I saw a 101 year old woman who could not get out of bed lifting weights so her arms would stay strong. There are very few good excuses not to do some form of physical exercise.

Yes you may hear some arguments of weight exercises being better than aerobics if you want to gain muscle and reduce fat. But this book is about losing weight. It is good if your goal is to replace fat with muscle, but our focus is solely on shedding pounds. I believe that any exercise that causes a sweat and that will burn calories is good.

Start out slow and develop a regular time and exercise routine. Then, next year, if you choose, you can do the more strenuous gym exercises. Remember, when you exercise you are not burning calories just during the exercise. Your metabolism will temporally increase so that you burn extra calories long after the exercise is over.

After you exercise be sure to pay attention to your feelings of hunger. Remember if you increase your food intake the calorie-burning effects of your exercise will be nullified.

You also may have to establish a habit of exercise using the information in the next two chapters.

> When it comes to eating right and exercising, there is no "I'll start tomorrow." Tomorrow is disease. — Terri Guillemets

Apples, grapefruit, pears, and broccoli have been shown to increase metabolism and thus assist in weight loss. Cold water fish such as salmon and tuna that are high in omega-3 fatty acids also tend to increase your metabolism.

Summary of the Chapter

In this chapter we learned that excessive eating is a disease and can lead to high blood pressure, diabetes, heart attack and other conditions. It is a major cause of premature death.

What causes us to be overweight is the consumption of processed carbohydrates. The resulting glucose quickly overloads our blood sugar levels. This causes our body to counteract the sugar rush with increased insulin production. The resulting fat is stored in our fat cells and this increases our weight.

The solution is to wean ourselves from eating processed carbohydrates. We can do this slowly but surely for a lasting lifetime of healthy weight.

Exercise is important, but for most people the majority of your weight loss will come from your improved eating (calories in) and not your (calories out) aerobic exercise.

Losing weight does not depend upon the new diet of the month or of the discovery of some pill. It does not depend upon your past, your vocation or your genes. People with your identical weight have permanently slimmed down using just habit change and subconscious mind control. You can lose weight by following the principles of **CAR** and **PREP** you will learn in chapters two and three.

> Obesity is a condition which proves that the Lord does not help those who help themselves and help themselves and help themselves. — Unknown

Almost all quick diets eventually result in regaining the lost weight. A slow change of lifestyle will result in permanent weight loss. You do not have to suddenly stop eating refined carbohydrates; you can cut down slowly and at your own pace. You will slowly but permanently change your eating and exercise habits.

You probably put your weight on over a period of many years. You still have many of the eating habits that allowed this weight to accumulate, so it stands to reason that it will take a long period of time to remove the weight and build new eating and exercise habits that will keep it from coming back. A quick weight loss diet will get some weight off but the track record shows that it will not keep it off.

There are two main parts to overeating. First is the habit of chewing and swallowing. This is a habit that is situated deep in our subconscious and comes from our human past when food was often very scarce. This habit can be modified.

Second is the refined carbohydrate (sugar) rush that gives you additional energy. It is both physiologically and physically addictive. When you slowly cut down the amount of refined carbohydrates you consume, you automatically reduce the power of your addiction.

Chapter Two
Habit Change

> Habit is a cable; we weave a thread each day, and at last we cannot break it.
> — Horace Mann (education reformist)

Humans resist change. Often it takes a disease, a crisis, or even a tragedy before we take a serious look at who we are and why we are addicted. But right now, you have the opportunity to decide to make the changes that will renew your life.

These next two chapters will give you the insights and techniques you need to change your habits and retake control of your mind. Many thousands of habits—both good and bad—control your everyday life. This book gives you the guidance you have been waiting for to help you change your negative behaviors.

A habit can be defined as an activity or behavior pattern that we repeat regularly. Habits are keys in our human ability that render us more advanced than animals. Psychologists also define habits as automatic behaviors triggered by situational cues. Habits make or break us to a far greater extent than we realize. The majority of our everyday actions are controlled by preprogrammed habits, which can either be positive or negative.

> The great power of habit for good and bad cannot be overestimated. — Theron Dumont

Habits make our brains more efficient, allowing us to avoid consciously thinking about routine tasks. Instead, we can concentrate on the newer or more challenging aspects of our current situation.

Habits also are very important factors in our ability to perform tasks quickly and without thinking. A simple example is wearing a seatbelt: most of us buckle up without thinking about it. A more complicated example is riding a bike. Learning to ride a bike requires a lot of attention to balance, and most of us fall a few times in the process of acquiring the skills. But once our subconscious brain takes over and converts a set of actions into an automatic routine, we can ride without ever consciously thinking about balance. Habits can make difficult or complicated things easy.

Habits can also be destructive. They can prevent us from considering why we do something or evaluating if we could do something in a better way. If we engage in a habit over a long enough time period, it becomes a part of who we are, and is therefore that much harder to overcome. You engage in habits subconsciously and often aren't aware that certain actions are actually regulated by a habit. As the saying goes, if you keep doing what you've been doing you'll keep getting what you've got.

Controlling habits is one of the few human skills that are known to produce an extraordinary list of positive benefits in almost all areas of your life. The good news is that you can change any bad habit and get positive benefits.

All of the things that can destroy your life are controlled by powerful habits. Using the instructions in this book, you can take that control back. You may think that willpower is all you need to change bad habits, but that isn't necessarily true. It works for some people, but just using your willpower to stop many habits is very difficult. One of my professors, when talking about willpower and habits, said that the average person believes he is above average. In other words, most people think they have above average willpower but in fact their willpower is just average. And most people need stronger than average willpower to change a strong habit.

> What you have to do and the way you have to do it is incredibly simple. Whether you are willing to do it, that's another matter.
> — Peter F. Drucker

If you think you have enough strength and willpower to stop a strong habit like smoking, then just do it. Many people can temporally stop some bad habits with their willpower. However, most of us are faced with a continuing conflict between the conscious mind that wants to stop smoking and the subconscious mind that wants the smoking habit to repeat itself again and again.

Day after day, month after month, most people will not have enough willpower to constantly fight their craving for smoking. Eventually, while our conscious mind is thinking about something else, some trigger will occur and cause our subconscious to pull us back into that particular bad habit. This could be a vicious circle with temporary victories followed by temporary and eventually long-term failure.

Instead of simply trying to control your bad habit with willpower, it is much easier to replace it with a better habit. To do this, you need to understand the operation of habits and the operation of your subconscious mind.

> It's the awareness of how you are stuck that lets you recover. — Fritz Perls

Sometimes people are afraid to make changes to their habits. It is the concept of "better to be with the problems I know than those that I do not know." If you have a pet dog, you have probably noticed that the dog is happy with its existing habits and does not like any change; at least until it gets accustomed to the new habit.

The good news about the following habit change system is that if you don't like the results, you can always use the same old smoking habits you used to have. There is no risk and you have nothing to lose by changing your habit.

> Nothing is impossible. The word itself says, "I'm possible!" — Audrey Hepburn

How habits work

The law of habit states that if you repeat an activity enough, it eventually forms a habit. Once the habit is established, your subconscious mind automatically responds in the same way every time a similar cue arises. For people who do not understand the subconscious mind, resisting it often takes more willpower than they have. Trying to fight or resist the habit usually just entrenches it even more strongly. The next chapter will provide more information on the subconscious mind control techniques that you will use to change your unwanted habits.

Chapter 2 Habit Change

> Men's natures are alike; it is their habits that separate them. — Confucius

Pavlov's famous experiment with dogs was one of the first scientific habit experiments that showed the influence of subconscious cues on actions. Pavlov rang a bell as the dogs were given food to eat. Saliva, produced in the mouth, helps in digestion of food. Naturally, the dogs salivated when they saw the food. After a number of bell and food repetitions, the bell was rung without any food but the dogs still salivated. Pavlov discovered that he created a habit in the dogs and the bell alone caused them to salivate.

During childhood, everyone acquires an assortment of various habits that affect them later in life. Some are good, and we want to keep them, but others are bad and negatively affect our lives. These habits are stored deep in our subconscious mind and we often have no awareness of where they first originated.

Like Pavlov's dogs, most of our habits begin without our conscious awareness. We do something and repeat it a number of times, and suddenly it is a habit that began without our awareness.

For example, one mechanical engineer I know was having difficulties on a project. He felt angry and frustrated, and after work used the whiskey, cheeseburger, and French fry method for coping with the stress. After a couple of months, this eating and drinking cycle became a habit, one which he performed every day.

Before he knew it, he was overweight and had a drinking problem. He was stuck in this cycle and felt powerless to make a change. He tried again and again to make a change, but he failed every time. He came to believe that he was powerless to change and was sentenced to a life of misery. Eventually, he just stopped trying.

These types of habits can be very difficult to break using only willpower, but you can change them. Your current circumstances and habits do not determine what you can be. Habits can be transformed using the science of habit and mind control described in this book.

> You will be the same person in five years as you are today except for the habits you change. — Professor Hal Cohen

In order to change a habit, the first thing you need to do is admit that there is some habit that you want to change. If you eat twice as much as you should and still think you are doing it for enjoyment, you will not try to change. In that case, reread the last chapter. If, after reading the eating chapter, you still think that you deserve all of that food, please pass this book on to someone else so they can change their life-destroying habits.

Cue, Action, Reward

> Motivation is what gets you started. Habit is what keeps you going. — Jim Ryun

Habits are created and can be changed with something called the habit cycle. The habit cycle begins with what's called the **cue**, which acts like an icon on your computer screen. When you click the icon, your computer triggers the associated program. It's the same with your brain when something triggers the **cue**. Then your brain turns on the associated routine to begin a particular habit cycle. For example, the smell of someone cooking food could set off a cue in your mind. A certain song could remind you of your first love. A certain touch could remind you of your mother's hug. A feeling of frustration, depression, helplessness, and other emotional issues could remind you that putting food in your mouth and chewing will make you feel better. These cues activate habit cycles and were probably setup accidentally and without your conscious awareness. Now they work automatically whenever the cue occurs.

Some cues can be avoided or changed, but some you can't change. When you take a work break, you may be in the habit of drinking a soft drink loaded with sugar to give you a boost. If that is your habit, you will automatically drink one whenever you take a break. If your habit is a sweet dessert after dinner, that habit **cue** will be there every time you eat dinner, and we all have to eat.

The habit cycle is as follows:

Cue ➔ Action ➔ Reward ➔➔➔➔ Habit Reset

After the cue comes the **action**, which is triggered by the cue. This is the physical action you perform. In the case of taking a work break, the action may be to drink a sugary soft drink and eat a candy bar. You can't change the cue because you need a break, but you can change the action. That is the first key of habit change science. You might find a substitute for the sugary soft drink and candy bar, such as chewing a stick of gum, eating an apple, or contacting a friend on your smart phone.

Finally comes the **reward**, where you get a psychological or physical reward. The reward is often receiving some type of desire such as pleasure or social acceptance in the work break group. Similarly, it could be relaxing by avoiding the unpleasantness of workplace frustration and impossible targets and requirements. Or it could be the acceptance from your group and avoiding their rejection. Cue, action, reward is a universal method to change any habit by replacing some part of that habit.

In our after dinner example, you get that comfortable, satisfying feeling that comes after a good meal and after a sweet dessert. The habit is then reinforced by the reward and reset waiting for the next cue to start the cycle again.

A good way to remember the habit cycle is by using the acronym **CAR**. This stands for **C**ue, **A**ction, and **R**eward. You can think of a car that requires you to steer it. Otherwise it will steer itself, causing an accident and possibly destroying your life. Habits are the same, and unless we learn how to steer and control them they will steer and control us.

> You must take personal responsibility. You cannot change the circumstances, the seasons, or the wind, but you can change yourself. — Jim Rohn

Habits are the foundation of many of our behaviors, and most of them were created subconsciously. Understanding the habit cycle allows us to be aware of these habits and gives us ways of changing them. We can use our understanding to create new routines that will change the habit and eliminate the bad or dangerous consequences of the habit cycle.

The great thing about habits is that once you establish or change them, they become practically effortless. It doesn't matter if you're tired or distracted, or have no willpower; the habit still takes over and fulfills your programming.

> Believe you can and you're halfway there.
> — Theodore Roosevelt

One very powerful key to changing habits is having faith in the possibility that it can be done. Some people might think that changing habits is too theoretical and might not work, but it has in fact worked for many millions of people. If you are dedicated to changing a bad habit, you can trust that this method will work for you just like it has for so many others. Once you understand that we can choose our habits, then you will realize that you can succeed in changing them. You can take responsibility for your own life. You can create your own habits.

> We first make our habits, and then our habits make us. — John Dryden

The thing about habits is that you are often unaware they control you. That is why the **CAR** idea is so important. To change a habit, you have to understand how that habit's **C**ue, **A**ction and **R**eward work. It may take some serious contemplation on your part, but the more knowledge you have about the **C**ues, **A**ctions, and **R**ewards of your habit, the easier it will be to change them.

Knowledge and purpose are all that is necessary to change a bad habit. Anyone can overcome habits if they truly want to.

> I can't change the direction of the wind, but I can adjust my sails to always reach my destination. — Jimmy Dean

The easiest link in the **CAR** habit to change is often the action. The other links can be changed or modified but are usually more difficult. Sometimes the cue can be modified if you discover that the cue is not what it seems, but the cue is sometimes more difficult to change since it often comes from our environment. For example, the delicious smells from the kitchen are often just there. Our action may be to get up and investigate the smells and have a bite to eat. The reward may be just an excuse to take a break from some disagreeable work. If this is the case, you can change the action and instead of food, take a break and maybe phone a friend, thereby changing the action and getting the same reward of a break but not becoming overweight.

It is important to understand the habit you choose to change. Break the habit down into the cue, action, and reward. Then think about the action and reward, and determine what rewards you are getting from the action you engage in. The next chapter will teach you how to control your subconscious mind.

> Successful people are simply those with success habits. — Brian Tracy

Make a list of each **cue** that makes you want to eat. Next to each **cue** write at least one way you can deal with or cope with that **cue**. Refer to the list while you are detoxing from your smoking habit.

If you can't change the cue, the next easiest link in the **CAR** habit to change is usually the **action**. The reward can be changed or modified but is often more difficult.

In some cases, the reward might be the temporary relief of your sweet food withdrawal. Removing this reward usually requires a period of enforced abstinence to allow your brain the time it needs to rewire itself and break the sweets addiction. Identification of the cue, action, and reward is necessary for the success of the habit change.

You don't need to keep eating the dangerous refined carbohydrates. Sweets can be comfortable and calming for your nerves, but if you slowly but surely reduce your refined carbohydrates you will break their hold on you. The problem is that you must then change your habits and subconscious mind programming to stay sugar free. Otherwise, you will be just like the millions who ride the roller coaster of diet and fail and diet and fail. So in addition to wanting to lose weight, you can get off the roller coaster if you reprogram your habits using **CAR**, as well as **PREP** and the seven step subconscious habit change sessions, both of which you will learn in the next chapter.

> Every grown-up man consists wholly of habits, although he is often unaware of it and even denies having any habits at all.
> — Gurdjieff

So now it's time to examine your eating habits. What are the reasons you overeat? Usually people will tell me that their reason for overeating is as comfort, to relieve their anxiety. Others say a sugary drink helps them concentrate, gives them a break, helps them relax, gives them a lift, helps their insecurity, et cetera.

As with habits, emotions are stored in your subconscious mind and can sometimes create feelings of anxiety or helplessness. People often cover up these helpless feelings with some comfort food their body does not really need.

When the comfort food is removed, those feelings sometimes return and a different addiction may take the food's place. If these helpless feelings are very strong, it may be necessary to discover their origins and work to eliminate or lessen their hold on you.

For many people the origins of these helpless feelings are already known. For others some serious self-examination may be needed. And some will need a few sessions with a professional therapist to get to the root of the problem.

One way to get an insight to the origins of your helplessness is to pay attention to your feelings when you first start to think about eating for comfort. You may feel inferior, unlovable, unworthy, ugly, gimpy, uneducated and so forth. Whatever it is, these are the issues that some people try to escape with eating behaviors. And if you don't examine these issues and work on them, you could possibly begin to escape them by becoming addicted to something else. If this happens to you, use the methods in chapter two to change the new addiction.

It is important to understand the various eating habits you choose to change. Break the habits down into their cue, action, and reward. Then think about the action and reward, and determine what rewards you are getting from the action you engage in. The next chapter will teach you how to control your subconscious mind. As we go through the following sections on various life-destroying eating habits, you will learn more about your individual habits.

> The greatest things ever done on Earth have been done little by little. — William Bryan

The Japanese have a concept called 'Kaizen.' Kaizen is a series of small steps for continuous improvement of something. Companies such as Toyota use it for quality, technology, productivity and company culture. However, it also works for changing your overeating habits.

History has shown us that long term habit change is most successful when you focus on smaller and more achievable goals. Often you need to break your habit down into small steps. In other words, instead of trying to throw a football the whole hundred yards for a touchdown, take it in baby steps. Throw a series of shorter, easier-to-catch passes and you'll still get into the end zone.

> I don't look to jump over 7-foot bars. I look around for 1-foot bars that I can step over. — Warren Buffett

Writers use a similar approach because most people just don't know where to start writing a long book. A large number of writers use the Swiss cheese method, which conceptually entails starting with a solid piece of cheese and taking out a small piece and then another and another until it is completely gone. Once you start at any point of the cheese, you have your foot in the door and you can move forward with writing your book.

> You don't have to be great to start, but you have to start to be great. — Zig Ziglar

Breaking up a large habit into a number of

smaller habits is an excellent way to overcome your natural resistance to change. Performing a smaller, more manageable habit change still gets you closer to your goal and has other benefits. In addition to beginning your motion towards your large goal, it increases your ability to change your habits. It is similar to lifting weights; you start out with a light weight and gradually progress up to heavier ones. With habit change, instead of building muscle, you are building the ability to conquer and control your habits.

> If you think small things don't matter, try spending the night in a room with a small mosquito. — Dalai Lama

In addition to compulsive comfort eating, you can do this with many other eating habits. Instead of using all your will power to eat less than 1,500 calories a day, you can just change your habit of eating ice cream for dessert. You can replace the ice cream with an apple. Then a few weeks later after the ice cream habit is successfully changed, you can change another eating habit. The reason this works so well is that learning to change smaller habits rewires you brain and makes it easier to change other habits.

Beliefs

> Champions don't do extraordinary things. They do ordinary things, but they do them without thinking - too fast for the other team to react. They follow the habits they've learned. — Tony Dungy, first black coach to win the Super Bowl

The most important thing about changing your habits is your belief that you can do it. An old quote that describes how this works is "You must believe it before you see it." In other words, you have to actually believe that the habit will change. If you do not believe it, then it is probable that nothing will change. You must be positive and know you can change. With a negative mindset, you will get negative results. Another saying is "if you believe you can change, you can. But if you believe you can't change, you can't."

There is every reason to believe that you can change any habit. In the real world, every single day, untold thousands of Americans change their bad habits and are no longer controlled by over-eating, nicotine, alcohol, drugs, and all the rest of the major life-destroying habits. These are people from every background and educational level. Smart people can change. Not as smart people can change. Rich people can change. Poor people can change. It doesn't matter who you are; everyone is capable of changing their habits. If all of those people can do it, then you can too. It takes some work, but if you are actually motivated to change and believe you can change, then you will. But you have to want it and believe in it. The good news is that through the techniques in this book, it's possible to change old habits and form new ones.

Motivation, belief, and the techniques in this book will allow you to bring about your change. The next chapter will provide you with techniques to heighten your will to change. It will explain how your mind works. It will give you techniques to redirect internal narratives so you can control yourself and change habits.

> Winning is not a sometime thing; it's an all-time thing. Winning is habit. Unfortunately, so is losing. — Vince Lombardi

Once you decide which part of your habit you are going to change, write it down. The act of writing gives additional power to your decision to change a habit. Put the note of your decision somewhere prominent, so that you see it every day. You may want to put it on your calendar or in your wallet or purse. In today's world, you can put it on your smart phone or tablet. I put my reminder in my iPad calendar so it appears every day. You should write down the habit change you want in detail in the present tense, as if it is already accomplished. The next chapter will have more information on why you want to write your reminder in the present tense.

Never make an exception to a habit that you recently changed. For example, I changed my habit of always walking down the grocery store candy aisle (and usually buying some candy) to never walking down it. Naturally, a few days later, I had the strongest urge to walk down the aisle, but my new habit prevailed.

A habit can be thought of as a piece of paper that

has been folded. Every time you refold the paper it has a tendency to fold along the same old crease. When we change the habit and make a new crease, the paper will initially easily fold along either the old or the new crease. At that point, a relapse to the old familiar behavioral habit can easily occur. After a week or two of folding in the new direction, the paper has a tendency to fold along the new crease.

It was the same with my candy aisle habit. After a few weeks, the urge to walk the candy aisle vanished. I just naturally avoided it and did not buy the candy that was a major factor in keeping my weight on.

> The great value of habits for good and bad cannot be overestimated. Habit is the deepest law of human nature. No one is stronger than their habits, because our habits either build up our strength or decrease it. — Theron Q. Dumont

You can't always avoid some eating cues or longings, so make a list of alternative actions you can do to distract yourself for a few minutes. A few of the many possible suggestions are:
- Get up and walk somewhere.
- Turn on some music.
- Phone or text a friend.
- Read a magazine or an Internet article.
- Go to a movie—but do not buy any food items from their concession stand.

> Habit is stronger than reason. — George Santayana

When a business wants its customers to habitually keep coming back, it uses a **CAR** model and adds one other phase to make the habit even more powerful. In addition to the cue, action and reward, they sometimes add investment. For example, if you use Facebook, your investment is in setting up your site with information, pictures and friends. Facebook then becomes a powerful habit that will cause you to sign onto your account more often.

Whenever someone starts a risky behavior, whether it's excessive food, cigarettes, drugs, alcohol, or something else entirely, they almost never realize that they are creating a habit and are going to be hooked. If they knew, it is unlikely they would ever allow themselves to become overweight and start the habit to begin with. But they didn't believe it would happen to them and now they have a problem. The most effective solution is to change the habit.

You don't have to be overweight. Your habits have made you that way, but you can control your habits and become a far better person than you are now.

> If you don't design your own life plan, chances are you'll fall into someone else's plan. And guess what they have planned for you? Not much. — Jim Rohn

John loved chocolate chip cookies, but he was overweight and knew he shouldn't eat them. Every night he needed something to snack on so he opened the cabinet and there was that new bag of cookies. He watched a bit of TV and finished the bag.

John's wife believed that the way to a man's heart is through his stomach and wanted to keep John happy. Every day she would put a new cookie bag in the cabinet. The next night he ate another bag.

John heard about the **CAR** method of habit control so he tried to replace the Action of eating the cookies with a raw carrot. But after eating the carrot, he ate the cookies anyway. John did not know about the **PREP** method you will learn in the next chapter, so he thought that maybe he could change the Cue. He had a long talk with his wife and the cookies stopped coming. John ate carrot sticks, but he still had a sweet tooth (sugar addiction) so he washed them down with a few soft drinks and got his sugar fix that way. Yes, John stumbled and fell back into his addiction, but that wasn't the end. If John knew about the **PREP** method in chapter three, he could have changed his cookie habit without drinking the soft drinks. Habit change is just the first part of the story. The next part is in chapter three. Below is a flow chart of the **CAR** method that John used:

Flow chart of John's process

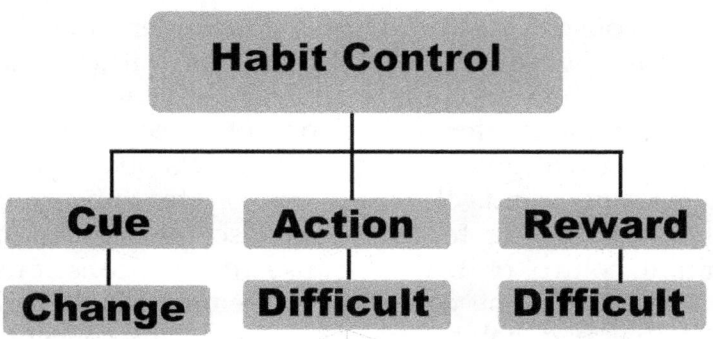

Summary of Chapter

> A habit is something you can do without thinking - which is why most of us have so many of them. — Frank Clark

In this chapter you learned that the vast majority of life is controlled by habits. Nothing is stronger than habits. Most of them are good habits and let you easily accomplish everyday tasks, such as driving a car while thinking of other things. However, some habits are detrimental, and you would like to get rid of them. Often you can just use willpower to delete bad habits, but sometimes you can't. You learned that particularly difficult habits are easier to change than delete. To change a habit, you have to study its components. These components are broken down into **C**ue, **A**ction, and **R**eward, or the acronym '**CAR**.'

There are some destructive habits that are resistant to the power of your conscious decision to change. This is because long-term habits are stored in your subconscious mind. Unless you understand the way your subconscious works, it is difficult to consciously change long-term, ingrained habits.

The next chapter focuses on subconscious mind control and will give you important facts about your subconscious mind. It will focus on teaching you methods of talking to your subconscious mind and regaining control of it. You can use your subconscious mind to change one of the components of **CAR** and defeat that bad habit. The most important concepts described in the next chapter are the acronym '**PREP**' and the seven step subconscious session to change habits. With these you will be able to use your conscious mind to change habits that are stored deep in your subconscious mind.

> Sow a thought, and you reap an act. Sow an act, and you reap a habit. Sow a habit, and you reap a character. Sow a character, and you reap a destiny. — Samuel Smiles

Chapter Three
Subconscious Mind Control

> Men occasionally stumble over the truth, but most pick themselves up and hurry off as if nothing has happened.
> — Winston Churchill

Everyone has an unbelievable power, but most people do not know about it. There are numerous things in life you cannot control, but you do have control over yourself and in particular your subconscious mind. You're about to discover the inner workings of your mind and how to control it to your advantage. It will be critical in your habit control, but it will also be important in thousands of other things in your life.

If you do not take charge of your subconscious mind, it will be your own worst enemy. It can easily override your willpower and best intentions. It can dictate your choices for you to blindly follow. It can make your life a living hell. But if you learn to control your subconscious mind, you can easily discipline it to do your bidding and help you reduce your weight.

> Your subconscious is a powerful and mysterious force which can either hold you back or help you move forward. Without its cooperation, your best goals will go unrealized; with its help, you are unbeatable. — Jenny Davidow

You're about to discover how to make your brain's subconscious computer work for you instead of against you. The power to do this is already within you. The simple techniques in this chapter will show you how to use your power and begin a brand new chapter in your life.

The power of your subconscious mind is far greater than you have ever imagined. It is the largest, most complex, and most powerful part of your mind. It has amazing powers, many of which we have still not discovered. There seems to be no limit to what our subconscious mind can do. And we only use a small fraction of our subconscious power.

Your subconscious is where your habits, as well as many other things, are stored. Subconscious mental programming is a wonderful technique that gives you the power to make changes that once seemed impossible. With this technique, you can change your destructive habits and regain control of your life. As you become more familiar with this subconscious technique, you will find that it becomes easier and easier to change all types of habits.

When I was eighteen years old, I took a course in self-defense taught by a really tough and experienced Korean War Special Forces veteran. In one lesson, I was very surprised how important it is to be aware of how my mind works. The particular lesson I refer to assumed someone was pointing a handgun at me. The trainers asked me what I would say. "Don't shoot" was my immediate response, and the rest of the class nodded in agreement.

"Wrong!" said my trainer. "It is extremely likely that the gunman is operating from his subconscious mind and this mind has difficulty understanding negative words or concepts such as 'don't.' All the subconscious hears is 'shoot.' It is far better to say something positive such as 'You win!' This puts the assailant at ease and removes the pressure from their trigger finger."

Next my trainer showed us how to disarm someone who was within arm's reach. He said, "Before you begin the moves that I will teach you, put the assailant in their conscious mind by asking a question." He recommended after saying, "You win," ask the assailant, "What do you want?" Even though I already knew what the assailant wanted, the purpose of this was to ask a question and cause a delay in the assailant's response time when I started the disarmament move. It turns out that the subconscious responds quickly and reflexively, like a computer or robot. The conscious mind can only think of one thing at a time; it takes a little longer to act because it is weighing the various options of the situation. By contrast, the subconscious mind is much faster. It can think of millions of different things at the same time so it arrives at a solution almost immediately and just does it.

We have two different kinds of minds. The conscious mind can decide which course of action is the most logical, but the conscious mind is also relatively slow. The subconscious mind can intuitively complete previously performed tasks, and it is much faster. You can reprogram your subconscious mind to create better ways to do these tasks.

The subconscious mind is the foundation or our

lives because it keeps us alive. It responds to threats much more quickly than our conscious mind and allows us to make automatic, split second decisions. It acts to escape dangerous animals or control our automobile to avoid a serious accident. And in addition to keeping us alive, the subconscious mind influences most of our everyday attitudes and decisions on almost everything. As the manager of our many habits, the subconscious mind controls what we eat, how much we eat, what we drink, the drugs we take, and the very health of our bodies. Our ability to regulate our subconscious mind makes all the difference between success and failure in life.

The subconscious mind uses over ninety percent of your brain, while the conscious mind takes less than ten percent. The subconscious mind can do things that the conscious mind has difficulty doing. For example, if you are playing tennis and your opponent is winning, you may want to change his subconscious concentration. One way to do this is to ask your opponent what he is doing differently to be playing so much better today. If he thinks about what he is doing during the next set, he will be in his conscious mind and he may be off his game since he can't react as well or as quickly from his conscious mind. You can try this out yourself by using your conscious mind to think about and do some simple task such as tie your shoe. Your subconscious mind can just do it all day, but your conscious mind takes longer to figure it out.

I have discovered that the mind behaves as if it had two parts. There is the conscious—or logical, rational—mind, and also the sub-conscious—or irrational, emotional, instinctive—mind. In almost every sport where quick reactions are essential, the good players are those who respond instinctively from the subconscious mind. The conscious mind can control the software that in turn controls the subconscious mind, but if the software did not come from you but instead was installed by others, the subconscious mind will perform its instructions and override your conscious mind. The physical brain is actually much more complicated, but the two minds concept is all you need to know to conquer and control your overeating habits.

In truth, the subconscious mind is the servant of the conscious mind, but it very often works in the opposite direction. Your conscious mind often goes to sleep and allows your subconscious mind to influence the decisions that dictate your life. Sometimes these decisions cause you to have various addictions that further control your life. When your subconscious mind works against your conscious mind, you will have problems. Unless you know the methods necessary to communicate with your subconscious mind, it will defeat your conscious mind. And the problems your subconscious creates will control your life.

> By learning the laws of mind, you can extract from that infinite storehouse within you everything you need in order to live life gloriously, joyously, and abundantly.
> — Joseph Murphy

Subconscious Mind

As I have stated, the subconscious mind can process information much more quickly than the conscious mind. When a cornerback intercepts a football pass, his subconscious mind is doing the equivalent of solving hugely complicated equations in just a few seconds. The football's velocity, drop speed, spin and wind direction are just some of the factors. If the linebacker used his conscious mind, the information would not be processed quickly enough and there wouldn't be an interception. The linebacker's years of practice in catching passes have forged the action into a subconscious habit and now it just all works automatically.

Many athletes rehearse their moves in their mind while they may be far away from the sports field, and possibly even while lying in bed. These rehearsals train their subconscious minds to create habits that perform certain actions as a reaction to certain moves by the opposition. Then when they get onto the field, they don't need to engage their conscious mind; the habits in their subconscious mind kick in automatically.

In golf, many top players imagine themselves making perfect swings and visualize the golf ball falling directly into the hole. These players are in effect changing bad playing habits and replacing them with winning habits. This does not have to be done on the green. Instead, they can practice in their own living rooms using just their minds. Researchers have determined that, even though the muscles do not move, the player's brain waves are identical regardless whether they are on the green or in the living room. When they get on the green, the habits they perfected in their mind magically work to improve their game.

> If we all did the things we are capable of doing, we would literally astound ourselves.
> — Thomas Edison

The subconscious mind also takes charge of all the things that happen automatically in your body, such as breathing, digesting food and so forth. While you sleep, it continues to remain alert and even generates your dreams. Additionally, it is an enormous hard drive that records the memories of everything that has happened in your life. It is also the seat of your instincts, emotions, creativity, beliefs and, most relevant to our purposes, your habits. It is the ideal place to make habit changes.

The subconscious remains only in the present time and not in the past or the future. The conscious mind can be in the past, present or future time. So when talking to your subconscious you must stay in the present tense; instead of saying, "I will be brave," you should say, "I am brave."

> Our subconscious minds have no sense of humor, play no jokes, and cannot tell the difference between reality and an imagined thought or image. What we continually think about eventually will manifest in our lives. — Robert Collier

The subconscious mind does not normally think with words. Instead, it prefers to use instinctive thoughts such as pictures and emotions. The use of pictures and emotions will allow your subconscious to more readily accept your conscious thoughts and programming. If you try to program the subconscious mind using the wrong words, it will reject the programming. Talking to your subconscious is similar to talking to a three-year-old child; you can't argue with it and you have to talk to it using simple concepts.

Your subconscious can't distinguish between what is real and what is unreal. No matter how unrealistic a concept is, if you can get your subconscious to believe the idea it will view that concept as a real fact. Then this new belief of your subconscious will be the new normal, and your life will now turn towards the direction of this new normal.

> For one who has conquered the mind, the mind is the best of friends; but for the one who has failed to do so, the mind will remain the greatest enemy.
> — Bhagavad Gita

As strange as it may seem, your choice of words and thoughts can make all the difference between success and failure with your control of your subconscious mind. But after you learn the language of your subconscious mind, you will be able to accomplish anything that you want. You will be able to take control of your life and change the habits that may now be destroying it.

When your subconscious mind accepts any idea, it begins to execute that idea. It is counter-intuitive but true that the subconscious mind accepts both real and unreal ideas equally. It does not argue like your conscious mind would. It is similar to a computer in that whatever it accepts, it believes. With computers, they say "garbage in makes garbage out," and it is the same with your subconscious mind. Our conscious mind sets limits for us, but our subconscious mind has no limits. It can do what we think is impossible. It can change our habits and free us from our addictions.

Many other people and events have already programmed your subconscious mind, but you are mostly unaware of this programming. You have a lot of garbage in your subconscious mind and you are being controlled by events in your childhood environment. It started when you were just a baby and continued through school and beyond. As a young child, your subconscious mind was aware of most of the things occurring around you, and stored them for future reference. Today, as an adult, this information often affects your thoughts, behaviors, and habits. Some of those habits can be very difficult to change if you don't learn the science of how to reprogram your subconscious mind. A prime example is your overeating habit, which you want to change but your subconscious wants to keep.

Your parents or other authorities may have wrongly told you that you were bad at something. That programmed it into your subconscious and to this day you probably still believe it. You were caught up in that belief, but what you didn't understand was it was someone else's belief that they gave to you. As a child, you had very little choice of what went into your subconscious. Schools, groups, friends, media, and governments continue to exert control of your subconscious habits, with the goal of making you into a more manageable subject.

The good news is that your addiction is probably not your fault. Your subconscious mind was programmed by others and it is likely that you had little or no control over the life-destroying habits that resulted. Your addiction is just the normal result of your subconscious mind dealing with various feelings of vulnerability that were programmed into it throughout your life. So do not blame yourself for the damaging habits that were put into your subconscious brain.

The even better news is that habits can be changed, and practically everyone has had to deal with some bad habits at one point in your life. You no longer have to live your life according to the subconscious programming installed when you were too young to realize its consequences. As an adult, you are free to change or at least update the habits that others have installed into your subconscious. This chapter will teach you how to do it.

> A man's subconscious self is not the ideal companion. It lurks for the greater part of his life in some dark den of its own, hidden away, and emerges only to taunt and deride and increase the misery of a miserable hour.
> —P. G. Wodehouse

The thoughts and images in your conscious mind become the messages your subconscious believes. Do not continue to think of yourself as a victim controlled by destructive habits that were implanted by others. You have the power to modify what you think, how you feel, and what you do. It is your attitude, and not your prior conditioning, that holds you back from being who you want to be. You can reprogram your subconscious and take control of your life. Make the decision to change the behavior you no longer want.

With the assistance of this book, you can change the addictions, negative self-image, vulnerabilities, and behaviors that automatically come from your subconscious mind. You can determine the habits that control you and choose to reprogram the undesirable thoughts that were put into your subconscious mind. Using the subconscious mind control methods in this book, you can replace those thoughts with the thoughts you want. You can change your life for the better.

> Why be just an average person? All the great achievements of history have been made by strong individuals who refused to consult statistics or to listen to those who could prove convincingly that what they wanted to do, and in fact ultimately did do, was completely impossible. — Eric Butterworth

Much of your childhood subconscious programming is positive, and you will want to keep it. However, a reasonable amount of it is negative, and this negative programming causes various bad habits and unhealthy states of mind that you will want to change. In order to change a habit, you need to use your conscious brain to reprogram your subconscious brain.

One of mankind's greatest discoveries is that you can alter your life by altering your subconscious mind. The only thing necessary for you to do is learn how to get your subconscious mind to accept your ideas and follow up with the subconscious habit change sessions described at the end of this chapter. Then the power of your subconscious mind will bring forth the changes you desire.

Any thoughts or beliefs that your subconscious has once learned can be unlearned. However, if you are not intentionally programming your subconscious with the correct thoughts, then it will still be programmed, but the programming will not be in your control. It may have been programmed by others, many years ago, and now it may not be beneficial to you. Understanding your subconscious is absolutely essential to successfully programming it.

Don't mistake this book's subconscious mind programming with simple affirmations. Sometimes affirmations will work, but often the desired habit change does not materialize, even after repeating a statement over and over for months. This is because of weak communication between our subconscious mind and conscious mind. It takes more than just saying some affirmation to make your subconscious believe it is true. You will have to learn the techniques to program your subconscious using the **PREP** method that I will explain later in this chapter.

> Begin to be now what you will be hereafter.
> — William James

To program your subconscious, it is essential that you perform the **PREP** method of subconscious mind control. Once your subconscious is reprogrammed, it will faithfully work day and night to bring about the requirements of its programming. If your subconscious is correctly programmed to believe that you should be a certain way, it will make it so. The amount of time that you believed your old programming makes no difference: your new program will take over from your old, obsolete program.

The subconscious mind works 24/7 to control all your body functions. It examines all the sensations (sights, sounds, etc.) coming to you from the outside world and then makes sense of them. It is the center of your emotions and inspirational thoughts. Depending on your subconscious programming, your view of the outside world is most likely different than mine. Unlike your conscious mind, which can only think of one thing at a time, your subconscious can think and do many things at the same time.

Your subconscious mind accepts and believes all thoughts correctly impressed upon it by your conscious mind. It is not able to distinguish the difference between truth and untruth. So if you absentmindedly say to yourself, "I'm too dumb" or "I'm too weak" or "I can't do this" and you believe it, then your subconscious will believe you and make sure you are unable to do it. If you tell your subconscious that you just can't seem to stop eating sugar products, you subconscious will believe you and prevent you from quitting.

Your subconscious mind will always accept your suggestions and will believe whatever is impressed upon it. It doesn't determine if something is good or bad. It doesn't determine if it is true of false. If you believe and think that you are unable to do something—and repeat the thought enough times—then you will not be able to do that thing.

> Whatever we plant in our subconscious mind and nourish with repetition and emotion will one day become a reality.
> — Earl Nightingale

When people greet you they often ask how you are doing. If you answer with something like "Not too good," "OK," or "I'm making it," your subconscious will be listening.

I personally always answer with emotion and in the positive. I answer with a positive word such as "great," "wonderful," "marvelous," or "groovy." My subconscious will be listening and direct my life in those directions. The only problem is that now some of my friends call me Mr. Groovy. At first look, this might be negative, but I just smile because even that helps program my subconscious mind.

Anyone who wants to change their bad habits and grow as a person should learn how to take control of their subconscious mind. When you do this, both your inner and outer worlds will change according to your wishes. If you follow the procedures and instructions of this book you will achieve the habit changes you previously thought to be impossible. But if you do not learn how to control your subconscious mind, then it will control you and your life will be as someone else has programmed. And it may not be to your liking.

When programming your subconscious, think in positives and not negatives. If you are trying to stop eating unhealthy food, do not focus on giving up or quitting this activity. All quitting thoughts are negatives. Instead, focus on what you want to do and not on what you don't want to do. In other words, you will focus on changing a habit rather than quitting it. You will tell your subconscious that when the habit **Cue** comes, it will do a different action that produces a different reward--such as chewing gum, for example. Instead of telling your subconscious that you will not eat unhealthy food any more, use all positives and tell it that you now eat only healthy food and that you are sugar free.

Your subconscious mind never sleeps and is always looking after you. Once your subconscious is reprogrammed, when the **Cue** comes, you will refrain from absentmindedly eating junk food because your subconscious will be alert and enforce your new habit. Like a computer, it will perform the programmed task, and you will not eat junk.

Your subconscious mind does not work in the past or future; it works in the now. Instead of using words such as "I will do something," use the present tense, which would be "I do something." Use the present tense and your subconscious mind will accept your conscious instructions as fact. Since your subconscious mind only accepts one concept at a time to be true, it will delete any conflicting beliefs and make your new belief its reality. At my university they called this cognitive dissonance. This occurs because of the fact that two contradictory concepts cannot both simultaneously occupy our subconscious. It is used extensively in advertising to sell you all manner of things.

> The more intensely we feel about an idea or a goal, the more assuredly the idea, buried deep in our subconscious, will direct us along the path to its fulfillment.
> — Earl Nightingale

What your subconscious mind believes and expects, your life will manifest. This is the key to changing the overeating habits that control your life. An example of this is the placebo effect. During World War Two, my father-in-law was a physician in the Pacific theater of war and often didn't have enough medicine to treat the huge number of causalities. He improvised and gave them a pill he said would ease their pain. Sometimes he even injected them with plain sterile water. Frequently the patient's pain improved despite the fact that the pill was just a placebo (a pill without any medication) with no physical effect on their condition. This happens because the subconscious mind believes that the pill or injection is real. It expects it will help to give them pain relief. Expecting pain relief, the subconscious mind blocks some of the pain.

Another difference between the minds is that the conscious mind tends to be more logical and the subconscious mind is more emotional. The conscious mind is the thinking mind, while the subconscious mind is the feeling mind.

> In the province of the mind, what one believes to be true either is true or becomes true. — John Lilly

Conscious Mind

Your consciousness is the logical part of your mind. It can analyze, criticize, judge, and choose between various possible courses of action. You will use your conscious mind to program your subconscious mind. Your subconscious mind has many automatic functions, such as keeping your heart beating and controlling your body's breathing. But in this book, we are not concerned with those functions; we are only concerned with how you can use your conscious mind to program your subconscious mind in order to change your unwanted habits. Your subconscious mind is also the seat of your emotions and the storehouse of memory where your habits are kept. We will use the repetition of emotions and pictures to change the habits performed by your subconscious mind.

If you or your environment conveyed unacceptable habits to your subconscious mind, the surest method of changing them is by communicating positive thoughts—properly directed, of course—to your subconscious. If done properly, your subconscious mind will accept these thoughts, thus forming new and healthy habits.

This is the same thing that many politicians and commercial advertisers do. They use emotions, suggestions, and repetition that your conscious mind may tune out, but your subconscious is always listening and often accepts the message uncritically. The advertisement is not aimed at your critical conscious mind but designed to influence your emotions on a deep, subconscious level. When they repeat the advertisement over and over, your conscious mind tunes it out. But your subconscious is always listening, and when it eventually believes the ad the ad becomes your truth.

In reprogramming your subconscious, it is also often advantageous to include harmonious emotions to give more power to the thoughts you use in programming. You know yourself that when strong emotional things happened to you as a child, you still remember them. Do you remember falling down and hurting yourself when you were learning to ride a bike? How about the time you excelled at something and were publically praised? You remember those things clearly, but you have long since forgotten other less emotional things. So we will often use emotions in concert with positive repetition to change habits more quickly and permanently. If you control your emotional state while you talk to your subconscious mind, you can more easily program it.

You need to understand that you can impress your thoughts upon your subconscious mind to change your habits. You can recreate your life and exchange bad habits for good ones. You can become the person you want to be. A few of us can make these changes using mere self-discipline, but most of us do not yet have that power over our minds. We must use subconscious mind control techniques to change our habitual ways of thinking and to modify the thoughts we no longer want. Eventually, as we have success in our programming, it will become easier and easier.

The law of the subconscious mind is that your programming can be changed by your conscious mind when you apply the procedures shown later in this chapter. You are like a commuter programmer: when you properly program your subconscious mind, it will do your bidding. If you let others program your subconscious mind, it will do their bidding.

One important concept you should accept is that you can change your subconscious thoughts. This change can cause your subconscious mind, and then your entire life, to improve dramatically. You should put aside all other concepts and dwell upon this fact until you have fixed it in your mind.

Do not listen to inner arguments against this idea. If a doubt comes to you, throw it aside. If you take your blinders off, even the darkest night will end and the sun will rise. You absolutely can change your thoughts and your life.

When you accept the power of your ability to control your thoughts, everything changes. It is phenomenal. The entire world seems to change. If weeds were planted in your subconscious mind, you can replace them with flowers. Yes, you can turn lemons into lemonade with just the power of your mind.

How to Control Your Subconscious

> Before I won my first Mr. Universe, I walked around the tournament like I owned it. I had won it so many times in my mind that there was no doubt I would win it.
> — Arnold Schwarzenegger

When you lose control of your habits and your life, you must reclaim it on your own; you will get little encouragement or advice from your friends. Don't expect anyone to help you. Just follow the instructions in this book and resolve to conquer your weaknesses. No one can do this for you. They can encourage you, they can give you examples of others who succeeded, and they can pray for you, but that is all. You must personally follow the procedures outlined in this chapter. You must do the work. Then and only then will you discover that when your habits are changed, new worlds and realities emerge.

> The secret of getting ahead is getting started.
> — Mark Twain

If you want a certain result in your habits, hold the image of the result in your mind during your subconscious habit change session, which I will soon describe. Keep your conscious mind positively certain that the correct result will come from your effort. Be sure to picture all the details of this result. After forming your thought, have absolute trust that your expectations are now reality. It is not enough that you want to believe it is possible to get a certain result. You must expect the result and know that it is real.

Your conscious mind can weigh ideas and accept or reject them, but your subconscious mind always believes what it is appropriately told. You do not have to prove or argue or fight about the ideas with your subconscious; it just accepts your conscious belief as true. Once your subconscious mind is programmed and believes something to be true, it controls your life accordingly until it is reprogrammed to believe something else.

The thoughts, pictures, and movies you program into your subconscious mind will become reality in your life. You should never think or speak of the change you want in any other way than as being absolutely sure that it is true and is happening. Be positive and your subconscious will accept the desired change as true.

> You can complain because roses have thorns, or you can rejoice because thorns have roses. — Unknown

Your first task to increase your control over your subconscious is to focus on and express your desire of what you want. Do you think it is best to change the **C**ue, the **A**ction or the **R**eward? You have to determine the habit changes you want very clearly and exactly. It should be a very lucid and very real knowledge. You should be able to envision what attaining the change would do for you. See yourself as already having achieved the change. The best place to change your subconscious mind is with your conscious mind. The **PREP** method shown below is the best way to proceed in reprogramming your subconscious mind.

PREP

One of my associates, Bill Malone, came up with the acronym **PREP**. It is a great way to remember the key **Prep**arations that are necessary to program your subconscious mind.

P is for positive. To program your subconscious mind, you have to send it information in a way that it understands. Your subconscious mind works with positive thoughts, pictures, emotions and feelings. It does not work at all with negative thinking. Remember that your subconscious computer has difficulty with negative words or concepts. It is not as discriminating as the conscious mind and will literally believe anything your conscious mind correctly tells it. The subconscious does not respond well to tentative thoughts such as "possibly" or "maybe." Give it positive, definite information.

People almost always use negatives when

thinking with their conscious mind. They will say something like "I don't want to be fat", or "I want to lose weight". The subconscious mind will not respond well to these statements. A positive statement would be something like "I am thin."

When I first heard about positive thinking, I thought it was a crock. But when I understood that it could be used as a method to program my subconscious mind, it suddenly made a lot of sense.

R is for repetition. You must repeat the instructions to your subconscious at least once a day for at least two months. This will be described further below.

E is for emotion and energy. Your subconscious mind pays particular value to a concept when you add strong emotions or passions to your programming words. Even advertisers and politicians use energy and emotions to capture your subconscious and get your sale or vote.

P is for picture. You should visualize that you already have the result you want. Think of it not as a change you want, but as a change you already have. Your mental pictures should be very specific and detailed. The more detailed, the better. For example, if you want to be sugar free during a work break, picture yourself as happily talking to your coworkers without a sugary soft drink can in your hand. You can even turn this picture into a mental movie.

If you want to lose weight, then envision yourself as the body shape that you want, wearing your new clothes. General concepts may not work, so picture yourself exactly as you want to be.

Your conscious mind must portray your desired results, not in the future, but in the present, as if the results have already happened. Instead of words like, "I want to," or "I will," use words like, "I am," or "I always." Hold your positive pictures and thoughts as already being the truth, and your uncritical subconscious will accept them.

The new or changed habit will quickly become your reality. If your conscious mind believes and trusts that you will change then your subconscious mind will also believe that and make it so. Picture your habit as already accomplished. The slogan "fake it until you make it" describes the process perfectly. Accept as fact that the changes you want are already reality. If your conscious mind believes it as fact, then soon your subconscious mind will also believe. "Believe it and you will see it," is an expression I heard often during my extensive studies.

Once your subconscious mind accepts your new programming as fact, it will bring this fact into reality and your habit will be changed. You will have reprogrammed your computer and it will now work with you instead of against you.

All belief begins in your will to believe. You cannot always instantaneously believe what you will to believe, but with time and effort your beliefs will change. This must be your first step toward changing your habits.

> The thing always happens that you really believe in and the belief in a thing makes it happen. — Frank Lloyd Wright

Your subconscious mind is like a garden, which may be intentionally cultivated or neglected and allowed to grow wild and controlled by weeds. But whether cultivated or neglected, it will grow. If the seeds are taken randomly from your environment, then an abundance of useless weeds will grow, often resulting in destructive habits. But you can tend the garden of your mind and weed out all the wrong, useless and destructive thoughts, replacing them with the flowers and fruits of useful and constructive thoughts. By pursuing this process you will discovers that you can change bad habits and actually become the director of your life.

A child's conscious mind develops more slowly than their subconscious mind, and habits acquired in childhood color your interpretation of your personal history. Consequently, you have misinterpreted many of the events that occurred in your early life. These distorted views of your life's events are now habits which continue to affect you today. For example, some adult may have tried to help by rescuing you from a hole you fell in. But the fall was painful and after the event you associate that particular adult with pain. The take-away there is that your past memories may not be accurate and, regardless of what you think your past was, you can use habit change and mind control to write your own future. You do not have to go back in time and correct that error; you just have to change your habits in the present time.

> Any thought that is passed on to the subconscious mind often enough and convincingly enough is finally accepted.
> — Robert Collier

Sometimes when you decide to change your life, you might have a fear of failure that could overwhelm your conscious desires. Again, be on guard not to think any negative thoughts lest they be accepted as true by your subconscious. Do not think about your problems, difficulties, or frustrations. Instead imagine your issues are already solved. Picture how the solution looks and how excited and happy you are that they have been solved so quickly.

The subconscious mind responds well to repetition. This is why to program your subconscious mind effectively, you must talk to it every single day. The subconscious will change to your needs if you send it instructions in a way that it understands. Everyone who puts in the effort of working on themselves will be successful.

No matter what you want, envision it clearly with detail. Picture yourself responding in a new way to those smells of food. Add feelings of joy and satisfaction when your changed habits obey your wishes.

The subconscious does not reason or judge how your conscious mind decides the truth. It just accepts and believes everything as factual and right. It works to bring your truth to life. The good news is that you can consciously overcome habits and control and rewrite your subconscious mind to work for you and not against you.

> Nothing great was ever achieved without enthusiasm. — Emerson

Set up at least one regular time every day for your subconscious programming session. This way you make these sessions a routine and then a habit. In the evening just before bedtime or when you first wake up are preferred, since at these times your subconscious is most susceptible to thoughts impressed upon it by your conscious mind. Another good time is just before or after a nap. Any regular quiet time of the day can work, but immediately before or after sleep works best. Many people have found that using an event, such as going to bed, works better than just using a clock time. In our busy lives, unexpected occurrences can disrupt our plans for programming at a specific time, but we go to bed virtually every day. The most important thing is to be regular and not to allow any excuse to keep you from your session.

Repeating something often enough causes your subconscious mind to believe it. This is the reason advertisers show the same commercial over and over.

At the end of your session, be grateful that your new reality is already here. This gratitude is perceived by your subconscious as further proof of what you want, and it will work harder to bring your desires to completion.

> Gratitude makes sense of our past, brings peace for today and creates a vision for tomorrow. — Melody Beatti

Reprogramming your subconscious is similar to building up your muscles at the gym. If you want to eventually lift 300 pounds, you might have to start with 30 pounds and work your way up. Training your subconscious is the same: you often have to start with just a part of the total change you eventually want. Every time you consciously reprogram your subconscious it becomes easier and easier.

> The difference between try and triumph is just a little umph! — Marvin Phillips

Seven Step Subconscious Session (SSSS)

Following are the instructions to program your subconscious mind. In the beginning, it might take you ten minutes or more. With a little practice, it will take seven minutes or less. Everyone who really wants to change a bad habit can find this small amount of time to completely change their life for the better. The best time to do this is just before going to sleep for the night or just after waking up in the morning. The transition between your waking state and your sleeping state naturally allows you better communication with your subconscious mind. Make sure you are in a place where it is unlikely that anything will disrupt your attention.

> If you accept the expectations of others, especially negative ones, then you never will change the outcome. — Michael Jordan

Seven Step Subconscious Session

Step 1. To begin your Seven Step Subconscious Session, write down the habit you want to change. Use the principles of talking to your subconscious mind and write it in a present, positive, and already true way. If you are working on overeating, an example would be "I am calm, relaxed, and refined carbohydrate free." Because of our formative years in elementary school, our subconscious elevates the written word above other thoughts and accepts it as truth. Handwriting works much better than typing.

Step 2. Sit or lie down, relax, and close your eyes. With your eyes still closed, roll them upward as if you were looking at the top of your forehead. This is a very important step that helps your conscious mind communicate and join with your subconscious mind.

Step 3. Inhale slowly, deeply drawing air in, and then exhale just as slowly. Let yourself relax as you exhale. Focus your attention on your breathing. Listen to the sound of the air going in and out of your body. Allow yourself to relax as you slowly breathe. Do this for three complete breaths. These three deep breaths increase your conscious control of your subconscious mind.

Step 4. Now, with your eyes still closed and still looking upward, speak or think the positive message you wrote down and want to implant into your subconscious. Say "I am calm, relaxed and refined carbohydrate free."

Change and adjust the words and images to control the habit of anything you are currently working on. Again, notice the message is in the present tense—"I am"—and not the future tense.

Step 5. Using sensory-rich details, visualize a picture or make a mental movie of your message. See yourself in all the detail you possibly can. Hear the sounds of your coworkers or friends talking. Smell the fresh outside air. Feel the happy thoughts of being smoke free. Try to use as many senses as possible to give substance to your vision. Whatever your goal is, see it as clearly as possible. Make the image crystal clear. Give your vision as much detail as you can. In your first session, there may not be a lot of detail, but as the days go by, you will be able to add more details to your vision.

Step 6. Add emotional content to the positive results. Recall something in your life that made you very happy. This may be a time when you achieved some huge success or some enormous win. It does not matter when it occurred but it must be something that made you feel genuinely happy. Relive the happy emotions of that wonderful past event. Re-experience the good feelings as if they were happening now. Recall your emotions as vividly as you possibly can. Now with those wonderful feelings, continue to repeat your subconscious statements you wrote down from step one.

Step 7. Relax and feel that the picture you created is now an actual fact. See yourself as already owning this habit change. Feel the thrill of your success in altering your habit. This is your new reality, so now open your eyes and give gratitude to the wonderful world that gave you this power. Gratitude is very important, since it signals to your subconscious that you have now completed this change—that it is real and is your actual present reality. Your subconscious will then find a way to fulfill this reality.

> Whatever the mind of man can conceive and believe, the mind of man can achieve.
> — Napoleon Hill

Upon completing your **Seven Step Subconscious Session**, take a minute or two to examine any ideas you might have had to improve your next session. For example, your subconscious mind may have given you feedback about something that might give you an insight about a cue, action or reward you are working on. If so, jot it down and adjust your next session to incorporate the new information.

The **Seven Step Subconscious Session** has linked happy feelings with change images and implanted them directly into your subconscious mind. This will cause your old habit to be replaced with your new visions. But one session is definitely not enough. Your old habit may have been in control for years and years, so it will take time to permanently change it. You have to be prepared to repeat these sessions for about two months. Everyone's time varies depending on the habit and your motivation. Some people can change a habit in a few weeks, while for others it may take six months. It also depends on the particular habit and your experience in habit change. If this is your first try, it may take longer. Additionally, a very strong habit will definitely take longer than a weak

Chapter 3 Subconscious Mind Control 101

habit. Also, as explained in the first chapter, you will need to detox your body so that your sugar consumption does not interfere with your **SSSS**, so changing your eating habit will definitely be one of the longer processes. Don't be discouraged, though; with patience and dedication, you can completely turn the habit around.

Notice that in this example, we used a **P**ositive statement, "I am calm, relaxed and refined carbohydrate free" instead of, "I will stop eating refined carbohydrates." The **R**epetition is daily for at least a month or more. The **E**motion is to recall something in your life that made you very happy. And the **P**icture is to see the eventual results as your present reality. See the lack of those carbohydrates in all the detail you possibly can. You can also include hearing and feeling senses. Your mental pictures should be very detailed; the more the better. It can even be a mental movie.

The methods here are for people whose desire for change is strong enough to overcome laziness and do the **S**even **S**tep **S**ubconscious **S**ession. A daily commitment is necessary. With this commitment, you must have an unwavering faith (fake it till you make it) that the habit is already changed and all you have to do is recognize it. Repetition is the key.

Again, what you have to do is form a distinct mental image of the goal you want. The goal comes from the habit you are changing. Also, hold fast to your purpose and be positive that your results will be forthcoming. Even if at first it takes more than two months, keep your positive attitude; if you do not believe, then your subconscious mind will not believe and it will resist change.

> There is no chance, no destiny, no fate that can circumvent or hinder or control the firm resolve of a determined soul.
> — Ella Wheeler Wilcox

Things that dominate our thoughts also dominate our beliefs. If you want to become sober, you most likely shouldn't make a study of types of wine and bourbon. Also, things are not brought into reality by thinking about their opposites.

Doubt or unbelief is as certain to start a movement away from your goals as faith and purpose are to start one toward them. Every minute you spend giving power to doubts and fears, every minute you spend in worry, every minute in which you are possessed by unbelief sets a current away from your goal of changing your habits.

> Destiny is not a matter of chance, it is a matter of choice; it is not a thing to be waited for. It is a thing to be achieved.
> — Winston Churchill

If you look at the majority of advertising and political campaigns that are directed at you, you will notice that very few of them use conscious, logical reasoning. They mostly use dumb advertisements that are filled with suggestions, dreams, emotions, and images that are implanted directly into your subconscious mind without any critical listening from your conscious mind. They have found that talking to your subconscious works and they spend many billions of dollars doing it. It works for them, and it will also work for you when you use the principles in this chapter.

Do not argue with your subconscious. Remember

that your subconscious is like a computer. You do not argue with your computer program. You know that your computer will not do something it was not programmed to do; you have to update the programming to get the functions you desire. It is the same with your subconscious.

> What lies behind us, and what lies before us are small matters compared to what lies within us. — Ralph Waldo Emerson

Use the instructions in this chapter to control your subconscious. Repeat the **SSSS** exercise once or twice a day. These seven steps may seem strange to you, but our subconscious mind is strange. We can either control it or it will control us. I choose control over my subconscious, and I hope you choose the same.

Your subconscious believes that there is something more official and real in the written word. In step one of the **S**even **S**tep **S**ubconscious **S**ession, you wrote down the habit you want to change as if it were already accomplished. Keep this paper in your wallet or purse until this habit change is established.

Computers and smart phones now have a number of programs that track and assist in forming habits. I believe that paper and pen work better, but some people prefer to do it digitally. If you are one of those people, do some research and find an app that works for you.

> There is a tide in the affairs of men, which, taken at the flood leads on to fortune. Omitted, all the voyage of their life is bound in shallows and in miseries.
> — William Shakespeare

You may think that change in your life should happen in the way that you expect, but often it's the opposite. You may try to change one part of your habit in a certain way but find that another part changed. Regardless of the exact change, your bad habit will have been fixed.

Do not be concerned about how things arrive; instead, hold onto your vision and follow the principles of subconscious mind control, and everything will end up in its place.

The power of belief is utterly fantastic. For all of recorded history, it was believed that humans were physically unable to run a four-minute mile. No one did until 1954. Then along came Roger Bannister, who not only believed it could be done but actually did it. That was great, but the amazing thing is that once people realized that four minutes was not a physical barrier but just a subconscious belief, everything changed. Within the next year, thirty other people had also ran a four-minute mile. Before 1954, no one could. By 1955, 31 people had.

For difficult habits, it sometimes helps to tell someone or some group about the change in your life. This is especially true for social people who are usually in groups or on their smart phones instead of by themselves. But never share your habit change progress with envious or negative people. Your subconscious will hear their negative response and possibly believe it. Only share your progress with positive, supportive people who will encourage you to continue your quest to conquer and control your habits.

When I first started writing, I shared my hopes and thoughts with someone who said that I would never be published, and he explained why. It bothered me for a while, but I overcame it and this is now my sixteenth book published by a variety of publishers.

> There is a track just waiting there for each of us, and once on it, doors will open that were not open before and would not open for anyone else. — Joseph Campbell

Most people are controlled by their subconscious and driven by the insecurities, vulnerabilities, and inadequacies in their life. They are passengers on the road of life and not drivers of the car. If you're not in the driving seat, you're being controlled or subjugated by the mental programs that you have accepted without even knowing it. You don't have to be subjugated by the mindless conditions that would rule and control you. If you use your conscious mind to reprogram your subconscious mind, you will no longer allow people or conditions to take advantage of you.

We all have worldly desires, and the subconscious directs us to do whatever it takes to fulfill these desires. You can rise above the programming and be free to choose your destiny.

Yes, it's easier to just go along with the crowd and do what they're doing, but you'll end up exactly like they are. You will be subjugated. You will be one of the masses; a cog in a wheel, a digit in a computer.

Psychology and money are the two main tools that people use to control you. But you don't need approval from others if it results in their control of you. Also, you don't need conventional status symbols, such as a millions of dollars or the finest sports car.

> Laugh and the world laughs with you; cry and you cry alone. — Unknown

A study was performed to demonstrate how controlled we are by social norms. The participants were divided into three groups. Group one was told that they would hear a joke and to behave as if it was a great joke. Groups two and three were not told anything. Groups one and two were put back together and after hearing a really bad joke group one laughed as they were told, and many in group two also began giggling and feeling surprisingly euphoric. As a control, group one was then told next time not to laugh at the joke. Groups one and three were put together and the same bad joke was told. No one laughed, and the joke bombed. It was the same joke but no one in group three laughed or thought it was a good joke. This is the same concept as the laugh track often played on TV comedy shows: the laughing from the TV show causes many viewers to be more prone to laugh.

You can use this concept by yourself; your behavior can create your emotions which are useful in the habit change exercise. Purposely tell yourself to smile and will you feel happier. Tense your muscles and pretend that you are vulnerable and in danger, and you become uptight and more focused on the present moment.

> It is never too late to be what you might have been. — George Eliot

I remember when I was young, a huge football player had words with me. Then he made a fist and took a swing at me. My subconscious mind took over and all I did was perform a very small action than had previously become a habit due to my training over and over in this precise move. I instinctively parried and, keeping contact with his arm, I pulled it. At the same time, I took a small step backward. He was off-balance due to the force of his swing, and I pulled him forward down hard. He hit the concrete ground with a very loud thump. He knocked himself out and didn't move. I looked around and saw he had a few friends, so I made a very quick exit. Due to many hundreds of repetitions, that one small step and pull became a habit in my subconscious mind and it saved me from what might have been a very dangerous situation.

> Magic is believing in yourself, if you can do that, you can make anything happen.
> — Johann Goethe

If you are just starting out with habit control and trying to make a huge change but are having difficulty, then take things one small step at a time. Just the smallest actions can make a big difference in your life. You don't have to go for the home run; just get on base.

> Nothing is particularly hard if you divide it into small jobs. — Henry Ford

In China, there is an old saying that "a journey of a thousand miles starts with a single step." Steve Jobs used this concept with his computers, iPods, iPads and iPhones. He came out with a great innovative product and continued to improve the original model, making it better and better.

Often, changing a big habit seems overpowering, so the solution is to break the habit down into a number of smaller changes. This develops the awareness that change is possible and strengthens your habit control. As you see the success of this concept, move ahead and change other habits until you complete all the changes you want.

> The great thing in the world is not so much where we stand as in what direction we are moving. — Oliver Wendell Holmes

After you change your unwanted unrefined carbohydrate habit, you may find that the psychological emotions your habit covered up are now exposed. It is good to pay attention to these exposed emotions because this gives you an opportunity for a deeper understanding of what issues drove your unwanted habit. Some people have found that these exposed emotions are redirected into other areas of their life. Fortunately, subconscious mind programming is also effective in eliminating the underlying issues and emotions that drove your habits in the first place. Alternatively, you may want to consult a professional to assist you with these issues.

Often times there are social habits that reinforce addictions. For example, if your social life revolves around a group where everyone eats a lot, you will need to change your social life and the places you frequent. Fortunately for you, your subconscious mind programming works on this as well as on the food addictions.

> Habit is habit, not to be thrown out the window by any man, but rather coaxed down the stairs one step at a time.
> — Mark Twain

Addictions are habits that are often associated with underlying emotions stored in your subconscious mind. Traumas, childhood abuse, neglect, violence, vulnerability, and emotional distress are some of the occurrences that produce these destructive habits. This is why we reprogram the subconscious and change these unwanted habits.

> Knowing is not enough. We must apply. Willing is not enough. We must do.
> — Johann Goethe

Summary of the Chapter

The only thing that could stop you from realizing the dream of changing your life-destroying smoking habit is procrastination. Procrastination means putting off something that you know you should do because of fear of change, avoiding confrontations, avoiding responsibility, or some other belief or feeling that drives you to maintain the status quo.

I am here to tell you that the habit change technology from chapter two combined with the subconscious mind control in this chapter is almost magic. It will lift your life to the next level where you will be free of the overeating habits that are slowly killing you. The only real thing that keeps you from taking action is you. You owe it to yourself to move beyond procrastination and take control of your life.

> I've failed over and over and over again in my life, and that is why I succeed.
> — Michael Jordan

Jane had a difficult boss at work, and every day

he criticized her. One of her coworkers was laid off and Jane was expected to take up the slack. Jane felt helpless and could barely make it through the day. She thought about quitting and getting another job, but it was a difficult job market, the economy was bad, and her pay was good. She knew that she was helplessly trapped. So to relax, she bought and ate comfort food in the form of an apple pie. They temporally took her mind off her problems and made Jane feel better, but she could actually feel her stomach getting bigger and knew she had to change her habits.

Jane examined the **CAR** of her habit and knew her boss wouldn't change so the **C**ue would be difficult to change. She also knew she needed some reward after work to make up for that terrible boss. So that left the **A**ction as the best bet to change. Her husband's health club had an elliptical machine, so on the way home she stopped in and used it for half an hour. It worked and she was able to skip the comfort food and take her anger and frustration out on the machine. On one unusually difficult day, however, her old **CAR** automatically drove her back to her old eating habit.

Jane knew it was time to use the **PREP** method to permanently change her action regarding those smokes. So for **P**ositive she decided on "To relax after work, I use the elliptical machine." For **R**epetition, she used every evening while lying in bed just before she went to sleep. Because of her anger at work, the **E**motions were easy. She just imagined that peace and serenity surrounded her when she walked on the machine. Finally, for the **P**icture, she envisioned herself as if in a movie, exercising on the elliptical machine and relaxing into a peaceful state.

She used this movie in her **S**even **S**tep **S**ubconscious **S**ession. First she wrote down that after work, she would use her elliptical machine to relax. Then every night as she was falling asleep, she rolled her eyes upward and slowly took seven breaths. She spoke the words she wrote on the paper and envisioned herself using the elliptical machine while being in a relaxed, peaceful state. She recalled the joy she felt when her father taught her to ride a bike and saw her actions as real and true. Then she gave thanks for the peace and comfort the elliptical machine gave her. In the days that followed, the old smoking habit was magically and permanently changed into the exercise habit.

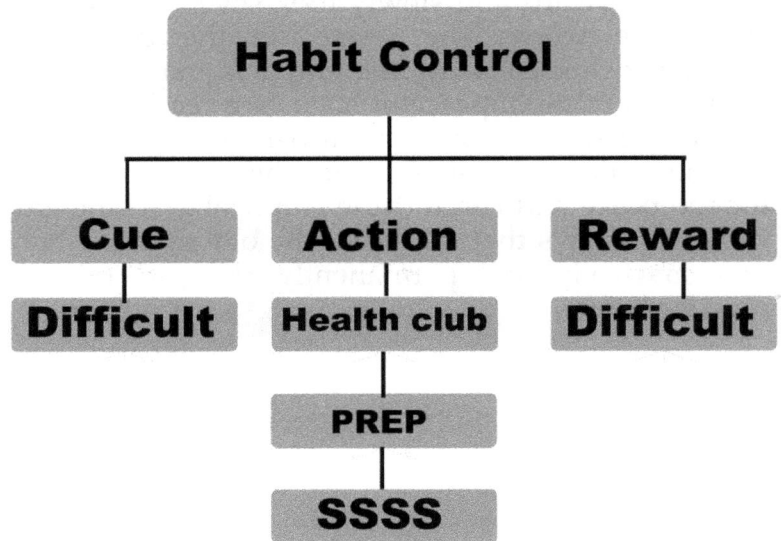

In this chapter, we learned the **PREP** technology. You can use **PREP** to change one of the components of **CAR** (from the previous chapter) and defeat the habit that is destroying your life.

<u>P is for positive</u>. Your subconscious computer has difficulty with negative words or concepts.
<u>R is for repetition</u>. You must repeat the instructions to your subconscious at least twice a day for at least a month or two.
<u>E is for emotion</u>. Your subconscious mind places particular value on a concept when you add strong emotions or passions to your programming words.
<u>P is for picture</u>. Your mental pictures should be very detailed. The more detailed the better.

"Fake it until you make it," is a memorable

slogan that describes the concept. Accept as fact that the changes you want are already reality. If your conscious mind believes it, then soon your subconscious mind will also believe. Once your subconscious mind accepts your new programming as fact, it will make that fact reality and your habit will be changed. You will have reprogrammed your computer, and it will now work with you instead of against you.

Do not be overly alarmed if you have a few relapses into your previous habit pattern. Just continue to faithfully do your subconscious mind reprogramming and you will soon be completely successful.

Conclusion

> Your resistance to change is likely to reach its peak when significant change is imminent. — George Leonard

In chapter two you learned that a habit is a **C**ue, an **A**ction, and a **R**eward. Many habits can be changed by just changing one of these three components. Often your willpower and the knowledge of how habits work is all you need.

However, overeating habits are difficult for most people to change with just willpower. Your conscious mind controls your willpower. If you decide to stop overeating by relying solely on willpower and some fast diet, you could easily fail. This is because in addition to your sugar addiction, your other eating habits are stored in your subconscious mind, which is stronger than your conscious mind. After a few weeks your willpower may wane and if you have a weak moment, you can easily return to your old way of eating. Habits are stored in your subconscious mind, and it is easiest to change them there.

To reprogram the subconscious, you need to know how to communicate with it. You learned to use **PREP** which stands for **P**ositive, **R**epetition, **E**motion, and **P**ictures. Then you learned how to perform your daily subconscious mind programming called the **S**even **S**tep **S**ubconscious **S**ystem.

In this book, I focused on weight control. However, there are literally thousands of additional habits that you may want to change. The **CAR**, **PREP**, and **SSSS** instructions will allow you to change them.

My other books in the Conquer and Control

series are located at the website:
ConquerandControl.com

They show you how to change many other habits using similar techniques. Additionally, I am writing other books to add to the Conquer and Control series.

Some of these habits are certainly minor, but you can still change them. For example, my physician told me to cut down my coffee drinking to eliminate my stomach pains. I easily went from eight cups a day down to just one. I probably could have done this with willpower, but it was easier to just let my subconscious mind take care of it.

> In any family, measles are less contagious than bad habits. — Mignon McLaughlin

If you are a student, you can change your study habits. If you fear public speaking, you can change that habit. The possibilities are endless. In the future, I will have more detailed information on changing some of these habits at:
http://www.conquerandcontrol.com.

Subconscious programming can also be used to switch off various abnormalities that cause pain. However, you should first consult your physician, because pain can be an indicator of a disease that requires treatment.

About The Author

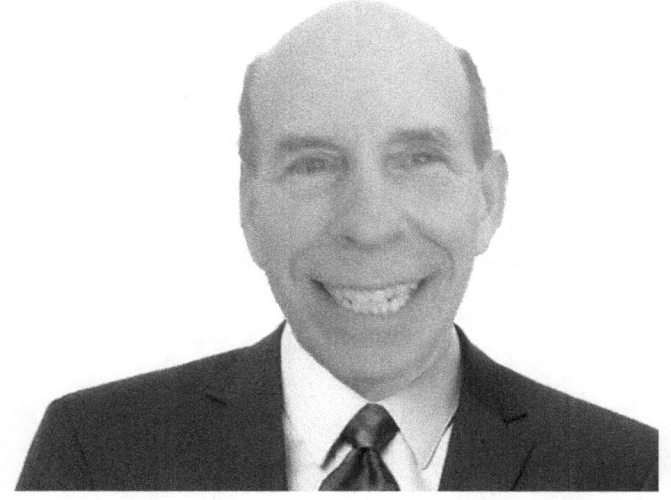

Alan Fensin began his career with Boeing and NASA in the early days of the American space program. He was a key member of the Apollo rocket design team that successfully put a man on the moon. As an electrical engineer, Alan helped design many of the critical elements used in the electrical system of the Saturn 5 moon–rocket. Returning to school in 1976, he earned an MBA from Tulane University, majoring in Behavior Analysis.

During the early 1990's, he discovered the *Conquer and Control* concepts and this system for using the subconscious mind to change unwanted habits. He believes that this knowledge changed his life, exposing and dealing with problems that had previously limited his growth.

He has been a lecturer and writer for the last twenty years.

www.ingramcontent.com/pod-product-compliance
Lightning Source LLC
Chambersburg PA
CBHW061449040426
42450CB00007B/1288